# Health Needs Assessment in Practice

# Health Needs Assessment in Practice

Edited by

**John Wright**

*Consultant in Epidemiology and Public Health Medicine,
Bradford Hospitals NHS Trust, Bradford, UK*

First published in 1998
by BMJ Books, BMA House, Tavistock Square,
London WC1H 9JR

**British Library Cataloguing in Publication Data**

A catalogue record for this book is available from the
British Library

ISBN 0-7279-1270-4

Typeset, printed and bound in Great Britain by
Latimer Trend & Company Ltd, Plymouth

# Contents

# Contributors

**Cam Donaldson**
Deputy Director
Health Economics Research Unit
Department of Public Health
University of Aberdeen
UK

**Therese Dowswell**
formerly Senior Research Fellow
Department of Psychology
University of Leeds
UK

**Stephen Gillam**
Director, Medical Development Programme
King's Fund
London
UK

**Stephen Harrison**
Reader in Health Policy and Politics
Nuffield Institute for Health
University of Leeds
UK

**Joanne Jordan**
Senior Research Fellow
Centre for Research in Primary Care
University of Leeds
UK

**Richard J Lilford**
Professor of Health Services Research
University of Birmingham and Director of Research and
Development
NHS Executive West Midlands Region
Birmingham
UK

**Maggie Mort**
Senior Research Fellow
Department of Management Studies
Lancaster University
UK

**Scott A Murray**
Senior Lecturer
Department of General Practice
University of Edinburgh
UK

**Anthony Scott**
Research Fellow
Health Economics Research Unit
Department of Public Health
University of Aberdeen
UK

**Andrew Stevens**
Professor of Public Health
Department of Public Health and Epidemiology
University of Birmingham
UK

**John Wilkinson**
Deputy Director of Public Health
North Yorkshire Health Authority
York
UK

**John Walley**
Senior Lecturer in International Public Health
Nuffield Institute for Health
University of Leeds
UK

**Rhys Williams**
Professor of Epidemiology and Public Health
Nuffield Institute for Health
University of Leeds
UK

**John Wright**
Consultant in Epidemiology and Public Health Medicine
Bradford Hospitals NHS Trust
Bradford Royal Infirmary
UK

# Preface

As health professionals we are taught how to respond to disease, but not about how to assess health. Although we try to fit the health needs of the patients that we see in hospital or primary care into neat medical pigeon holes, they may require much more complex solutions which recognise the wider influences on health. As for the patients we do not see, their health needs may be just as important, and yet go unheard.

Health reforms world wide have led to greater demands for hospitals and primary care teams to provide health services that meet the needs of their local populations rather than services just developed in response to the personal interests of a few individuals. Changing patient expectations as health consumers have provided extra impetus. As health professionals we now have a responsibility to ensure that limited resources are used to provide the most appropriate and effective health care to meet patients' needs. The challenge is how we can best assess these needs in practice.

This book brings together a wealth of experience in the field to describe the practical approaches to assessing health needs, and how the results can be used effectively to improve the health of local populations. Many of the techniques of community appraisals used in needs assessment originate from experience in developing countries, and lessons from this experience are included. Assessing health is not easy to describe in eight chapters, but I hope that this book provides a clear focus for future work. I am very grateful to all the contributors who have shared their enthusiasm and commitment to this project and would like to thank John Bibby, Dee Kyle, Sheila Webb, Antony Zwi and Margaret Haigh for their advice and support.

John Wright

# 1 The development and importance of health needs assessment

JOHN WRIGHT,
RHYS WILLIAMS, and
JOHN WILKINSON

Most doctors are used to assessing the health needs of their individual patients. Professional training and clinical experience teach us a systematic approach to this assessment before we commence a treatment which we believe to be effective. Such a systematic approach has often been missing when it comes to assessing the health needs of a local or practice population.

The health needs of individual patients coming through the consulting room door may not reflect the wider health needs of the community. If people have a health problem that they believe cannot be helped by the health service, then they will not attend. For example, many people with angina or multiple sclerosis are not known to either their local general practitioner or hospital specialist.[1,2] Other groups of patients who may need health care but do not demand it include homeless people and those with chronic mental illness.

The distinction between individual needs and the wider needs of the community should be taken into consideration when local health services are being planned. If they are ignored there is a danger of a top-down approach to providing health services that relies too heavily on what a few people perceive to be the needs of the population rather than what they actually are.

Health needs assessment is a new phrase to describe the development and refinement of well established approaches to understanding the needs of a local population. In the nineteenth

1

century the first Medical Officers for Health were responsible for assessing the needs of their local populations. More recently in the 1970s the Resource Allocation Working Party assessed relative health needs on the basis of standardised mortality ratios and socioeconomic deprivation in different populations, and used this formula to recommend fairer redistribution of health service resources.[3] *The Health of the Nation* initiative was a government attempt to assess national health needs and determine priorities for improving health.[4] The phrase has come to mean an objective and valid method of tailoring health services, an evidence based approach to commissioning and planning health services.

Although health needs assessments have traditionally been undertaken by public health professionals looking at their local population, these needs should be paramount to all health professionals. Both hospital and primary care teams should aim to develop services to match their local population's needs. Combining population needs assessment with personal knowledge of patients' needs may help to meet this goal.[5]

## Why has needs assessment become important?

The costs of health care are rising. Over the last 30 years health care expenditures have risen much faster than the cost increases reported in other sectors of the economy, and health care is now one of the largest sectors in most developed countries.[6] Medical advances and demographic changes will continue the upward pressure on costs.[7]

At the same time there are limited resources available for health care. Many individuals have inequitable access to adequate health care, and many governments are unable to provide it universally. In addition there is a large variation in health care availability and use by geographical area and health care setting.[8] The availability of this health care tends to be inversely related to the need of the population served.[9]

Consumerism is also an increasing force for change. Public expectations have led to greater concerns about the quality of the services they receive, from access and equity to appropriateness and effectiveness.

These factors have been a trigger for health service reforms in both developed and developing countries. In the UK these reforms resulted in the separation of the responsibility for financing health care from its provision, and establishment of a purchasing role for health authorities and general practitioners. Health authorities had greater opportunities to try to tailor local services to their own populations, and the 1990 National Health Service Act made it a requirement for health authorities to assess health needs of their populations, and to use these assessments to set priorities to improve the health of their local population.[10,11] This has been reinforced by more recent work on inequalities in health, suggesting that health authorities should undertake "equity audits" to determine if health care resources are being used in accordance with need.[12]

At a primary care level, through fundholding, locality commissioning, and total purchasing projects, general practitioners became more central to strategic planning and development of health services. With this increased commissioning power came the increased expectations from patients and politicians that decision-making would reflect local and national priorities, promoting effective and equitable care on the basis of need.[13] The new Labour government has committed itself to ensuring access to treatment according to "need and need alone", and the key functions of Primary Care Groups will be to plan, commission, and monitor local health services to meet identified local needs.[14,15]

## Needs

Doctors, sociologists, philosophers, and economists all have different views of what needs are.[16–20] In recognition of the scarcity of resources available to meet these needs, differentiation of health needs is often made into needs, demands, and supply (Figure 1.1).

- *Need* in health care is commonly defined as the capacity to benefit. If health needs are to be identified then there should be an effective intervention available to meet these needs and improve health. There will be no benefit from an intervention that is not effective or there are no resources available to resource.
- *Demand* is what patients ask for and the needs that most doctors encounter. General practitioners have a key role as gatekeepers in controlling this demand, and waiting lists become a surrogate marker and an influence on this demand. Demand from patients for a service can be dependent on the characteristics of the patient or the media interest in the service. Demand can also be

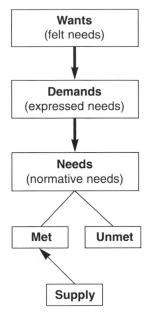

*Figure 1.1    Different aspects of needs.*

supply-induced. For example, geographical variation in hospital admission rates is explained more by the supply of hospital beds than indicators of mortality.[21-22] Referral rates by general practitioners owe more to the characteristics of individual doctors than the health of their populations.[23]

- *Supply* is the health care provided. This will depend on the interests of health professionals, the priorities of politicians and the amount of money available. National health technology assessment programmes have developed in recognition of the importance of assessing the supply of new services and treatments before their widespread introduction.

Need, demand and supply overlap and this relationship is important to consider when health needs are assessed (Figure 1.2).[20]

## Health needs

The World Health Organisation's definition of health is often used: "Health is a state of complete physical, psychological and

4

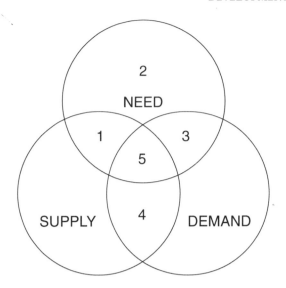

*Figure 1.2  Relationship between need, supply, and demand.*
*(1) Need and supply but **no** demand (e.g. health promotion, some screening).*
*(2) Need but **no** supply or demand (e.g. treatment of child abusers).*
*(3) Need and demand but **no** supply (e.g. termination of pregnancy, waiting lists).*
*(4) Supply and demand but **no** need (e.g. antibiotics for viral upper respiratory tract infections).*
*(5) Ideal relationship between need, supply, and demand.*
*Adapted with permission from Stevens A, Raftery J, eds.* Health Care Needs Assessment, the epidemiologically based needs assessment reviews. *Oxford: Radcliffe Medical Press, Vol. 1, 1994.*

social well-being and not simply the absence of disease or infirmity." A more romantic definition would be Freud's: "Health is the ability to work and to love."

- *Health care needs* are those that can benefit from health care (health education, disease prevention, diagnosis, treatment, rehabilitation, terminal care). Most doctors will consider needs in terms of health care services which they can supply. Patients, however, may have a different view of what would make them healthier, for example a job, a bus route to the hospital or health centre, or decent housing.

- *Health needs* incorporates the wider social and environmental determinants of health, such as deprivation, housing, diet, education, employment. This wider definition allows us to look beyond the confines of the medical model based on health

---

**Box 1.1    Influences on health**

- Environment: housing, education, socioeconomic status, pollution
- Behaviour: diet, smoking, exercise
- Genes: inherited health potential
- Health care: including primary, secondary, and tertiary prevention

---

services, to the wider influences on health (Box 1.1). Health needs of a population will be constantly changing, and many will not be so amenable to medical intervention.

## Health Needs Assessment

Assessment of health needs is not simply a process of listening to patients or relying on personal experience. It is a systematic method of identifying unmet health and health care needs of a population, and making changes to meet these unmet needs. It involves an epidemiological and qualitative approach to determining priorities, which incorporates clinical and cost effectiveness and patients' perspectives. This approach must balance clinical, ethical, and economic considerations of need, that is what should be done, what can be done, and what can be afforded.[24]

Health needs assessment should not just be a method of measuring ill health, as this assumes that something can be done to tackle it. Incorporating the concept of a capacity to benefit introduces the importance of effectiveness of health interventions, and attempts to make explicit what benefits are being pursued. Economists argue that the capacity to benefit is always going to be greater than available resources, and that health needs assessment should also incorporate questions of priority setting,[25] suggesting that many needs assessments are simply distractions from the difficult decisions of rationing.[26]

For individual practices and health professionals, health needs assessment provides the opportunity for:

- describing the patterns of disease in the local population and the differences from district, regional, or national disease patterns;

- learning more about the needs and priorities of their patients and the local population;
- highlighting the areas of unmet needs and providing a clear set of objectives to work towards to meet these needs;
- deciding rationally how to use resources to improve their local population's health in the most effective and efficient way;
- influencing policy, interagency collaboration, or research and development priorities.

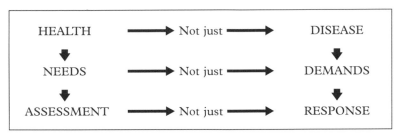

Importantly it also provides a method of monitoring and promoting equity in the provision and use of health services and addressing inequalities in health.[27,28]

The importance of assessing health needs rather than reacting to health demands is widely recognised and there are many examples of needs assessment in primary and secondary care.[29–31]

There is no easy, quick-fix recipe for health needs assessment. Different topics will require different approaches. This may involve a combination of qualitative and quantitative research methods to collect original information, or adapting and transferring what is already known or available.

The stimulus for these assessments is often the personal interest of an individual or the availability of new funding for the development of health services. However, they should also be prompted by the importance of the health problem (in terms of frequency, impact, or cost), the occurrence of critical incidents (the death of a patient turned away from a full intensive care unit), evidence of effectiveness of an intervention, or publication of new research findings about the burden of a disease.

Some needs assessments have been more successful than others. Projects may fail for the reasons below.[30,32,33]

(1) *A lack of understanding of what is involved in assessing health needs and how it should be undertaken.* Educational strategies

7

can improve the understanding and necessary skills of health professionals, and local public health teams can provide valuable support and guidance. Commonsense can be a more important asset than detailed methodological understanding.[34] Starting with a simple and well defined health topic can provide experience and encourage success.

(2) *A lack of time, resources, or commitment.* The time and resources required can be small when shared between a team of professionals, and such sharing has the potential to be team-building. Involvement of other organisations such as social services, local authorities, or voluntary groups can provide similar advantages and encourage multiagency working.

Integration of needs assessment into audit and education can also provide better use of scarce time. Such investment of time and effort is likely to become increasingly necessary in order to justify extra resources.

(3) *Failure to integrate the results with planning and purchasing intentions to produce change.* The planning cycle should begin with the assessment of need.[27] Objectives must be clearly defined (see box below) and relevant stakeholders or agencies (Figure 1.3) appropriately involved. Although such an assessment may produce a multitude of needs, criteria can be used to prioritise these needs; for example, the importance of problem in terms of frequency or severity; the evidence of effectiveness of interventions, or the feasibility for change.

---

### Box 1.2   A framework of questions to ask when assessing health needs

- What is the problem?
- What is the size and nature of the problem?
- What are the current services?
- What do patients want?
- What are the most appropriate and effective (clinical and cost) solutions?
- What are the resource implications?
- What are the outcomes to evaluate change and the criteria to audit success?

---

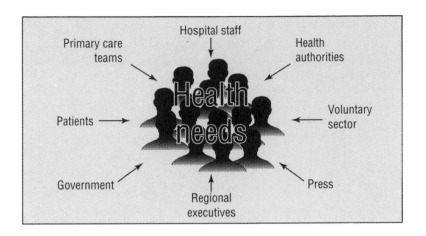

*Figure 1.3   Contributors to needs assessment.*

Needs assessments that do not include sufficient attention to implementation will become little more than academic or public relations exercises.

This book will describe the different approaches to assessing health needs, how to identify topics for health needs assessments, which practical approaches can be taken, and how the results can be used effectively to improve the health of local populations. It will give examples of needs assessment from primary care but will also cover the specific problems of needs assessment for hard-to-reach groups. Many of the techniques of community appraisals used in needs assessment originate from experience in developing countries and some of the lessons from this experience will be described.

## Acknowledgements

We are grateful to John Bibby, Sheila Webb, and Dee Kyle for their valuable contributions and to Margaret Haigh for her secretarial support.

9

## Summary points

- Health needs assessment is the systematic approach to ensuring that the health service uses its resources to improve the health of the population in the most efficient way.
- It involves epidemiological, qualitative and comparative methods to:
  - describe health problems of a population;
  - identify inequalities in health and access to services;
  - determine priorities for the most effective use of resources.
- Health needs may be those needs which can benefit from health care or from wider social and environmental changes.
- For health needs assessments to be successful there must be a practical understanding of what is involved, the time and resources necessary to undertake assessments, and sufficient integration of the results into planning and commissioning of local services.

# References

1 Smith R. Rationing: the search for sunlight (editorial). *BMJ* 1991;**303**:1561–2.
2 Ford HL, Gerry E, Airey CM, Johnson MH, Williams DRR. The prevalence of multiple sclerosis in the Leeds District. *J Neurol Neurosurg Psychiatry* 1998 (in press).
3 Department of Health and Social Security. *Sharing resources for health in England: report of the Resource Allocation Working Party.* London: HMSO, 1976.
4 Department of Health. *The Health of the Nation: a strategy for health in England* (CM 1986). London: HMSO, 1992.
5 Shanks J, Kheraj S, Fish S. Better ways of assessing health needs in primary care. *BMJ* 1995;**310**:480–1.
6 Organisation for Economic Cooperation and Development. *Health care systems in transition: the search for efficiency.* (Social Policy Studies No.7). Paris: OECD, 1990.
7 Harrison A, Dixon J, New B, Judge K. Funding the NHS. Can the NHS cope in future. *BMJ* 1997;**314**:139–42.
8 Anderson TV, Mooney G. *The challenge of medical practice variations.* London: Macmillan Press, 1990.
9 Tudor Hart J. The inverse care law. *Lancet* 1971;**I**:405–12.
10 Department of Health. *Working for patients* (CM 555). London: HMSO, 1989.
11 National Health Service Management Executive (1991). *Assessing health care needs.* DHA project discussion paper. Leeds: NHSME, 1991.
12 Variations Subgroup of the Chief Medical Officer's Health of the Nation Working Group. *Variations in health. What can the Department of Health and the NHS do?* London: Department of Health, 1995.
13 National Health Service Executive. *An accountability framework for GP fundholding: towards a primary care led NHS.* EL(94)54 Leeds: NHSE, 1994.
14 Secretary of State for Scotland. *Designed to Care.* Edinburgh: Department of Home and Health. Scottish Office. 1997.

15 *The New NHS*. London: Stationery Office, 1997. (Cm 3807)
16 Culyer AJ. *Need and the National Health Service*. London: Martin Robertson, 1976.
17 Bradshaw J. A taxonomy of social need. In: McLachlan G, ed. *Problems and progress in medical care*. 7th series. London: Oxford University Press, 1972.
18 Frankel S. Health needs, health-care requirements and the myth of infinite demand. *Lancet* 1991;337:1588–9.
19 Williams A. Priorities not needs. In: Corden A, Robertson G, Tolley K, eds. *Meeting needs*. Aldershot: Avebury Gower, 1992.
20 Stevens A, Gabbay J. Needs assessment needs assessment. . . . *Health Trends* 1991;23:20–23.
21 Feldstein MS. Effects of differences in hospital bed scarcity on type of use. *BMJ* 1964;2:562–5.
22 Kirkup B, Forster D. How will health needs be measured in districts? Implications of variations in hospital use. *J Public Health Med* 1990;12:45–50.
23 Wilkin D. Patterns of referral: explaining variation. In Roland M, Coulter A, eds. *Hospital referrals*. Oxford: Oxford University Press 1992.
24 Black D. *A doctor looks at health economics*. Office of Health Economics Annual Lecture. London: OHE, 1994.
25 Donaldson C, Mooney G. Needs assessment, priority setting, and contracts for health care: an economic view. *BMJ* 1991;303:31529–30.
26 Mooney G. *Key issues in health economics*. Hemel Hempstead: Harvester Wheatsheaf, 1994.
27 Womersley J, McCauley D. Tailoring health services to the needs of individual communities. *J Publ Health Med* 1987;41:190–5.
28 Majeed FA, Chaturvedi N, Reading R, Ben-Shlomo Y. Monitoring and promoting equity in primary and secondary care. *BMJ* 1994;308:1426–9.
29 Gillam SJ, Murray SA. *Needs assessment in general practice*. Occasional paper 73. Royal College of General Practitioners. London, 1996.
30 Jordan J, Wright J, Wilkinson J, Williams DRR. *Health needs assessment in primary care: a study of the understanding and experience in three districts*. Leeds: Nuffield Institute for Health, 1996.
31 Stevens A, Raftery J, eds. *Health care needs assessment – the epidemiologically based needs assessment reviews*. Oxford: Radcliffe Medical Press, 1994.
32 London Health Economics Consortium. *Local health and the vocal community, a review of developing practice in community based health needs assessment*. London: London Primary Health Care Forum, 1996.
33 Jordan J, Wright J. Making sense of health needs assessment. *Brit J Gen Pract* 1997;48:695–6.
34 Gillam S. Assessing the health care needs of populations – the general practitioner's contribution (Editorial). *Br J Gen Pract* 1992;42:404–5.

11

# 2 Epidemiological issues in health needs assessment

RHYS WILLIAMS and JOHN WRIGHT

## What is the "epidemiological approach" to health needs assessment?

Chapter 1 explained the importance of health needs assessment in the context of planning and delivering health care to populations. The "epidemiological approach" to health needs assessment was mentioned. This is the traditional public health approach of describing need in relation to specific health problems using estimates of the incidence, prevalence, and other surrogates of health impact derived from studies carried out locally or elsewhere. It has been be extended[1] to the consideration, alongside these measures, of the ways in which existing services are delivered and the effectiveness and cost effectiveness of interventions intended to meet the needs thus described (Figure 2.1). This is a logical

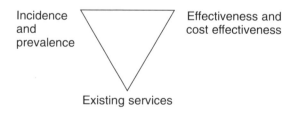

Incidence and prevalence

Effectiveness and cost effectiveness

Existing services

*Figure 2.1 Components of health needs assessment. Adapted with permission from Stevens A, Raftery J, eds. Health Care Needs Assessment: the epidemiologically based needs assessment reviews. Oxford Medical Press, Vol. 1, 1994.*

extension as there is little point in estimating the burden of ill health (except for the prioritisation of future research) if nothing can be done to reduce it.

Epidemiology has been defined[2] as "the study of the distribution and determinants of health-related states or events in specific populations and the application of this study to control of health problems". It tends, for the most part, to use the "medical model" of health need that is viewed in terms of the occurrence of specific diseases and health-related states rather than client groups. Descriptive epidemiology (as opposed to analytical epidemiology – the investigation of the determinants of health-related states or events) describes the occurrence of disease in terms of person, place, and time.

- **Person** – Who are the affected people (in terms of their age, gender, occupation, socioeconomic group etc.)?
- **Place** – Where are they when they get diseases and in what way do prevalence and incidence vary geographically (locally, regionally, nationally, or internationally)?
- **Time** – When do people get diseases, does this vary by, for example, season, and how is disease occurrence changing over time?

Important principles when an epidemiological survey is made are listed in the box below.

## Case definition

The usual starting point for any epidemiologically based needs assessment is the question – what is a case? Epidemiologists place great importance on case definition although, for a thorough health needs assessment, simple case definitions usually need to be expanded to include valid measures of severity.

Cases may possess relatively clear characteristics which separate them from those who are not cases. Examples are those with the florid symptoms or signs of hypertension, asthma, or diabetes. However, in most conditions, including these three, individuals are encountered who are close to the borderline between normality and abnormality (Figure 2.2). For these, internationally agreed criteria are required and are available.[3-5]

---

### Box 2.1  Important principles involved in the undertaking of an epidemiological survey

Routine sources can provide only limited descriptions of disease. In order to provide more details, special surveys may be required. There are two main types of descriptive survey: *prevalence* or cross-sectional surveys, and *longitudinal* surveys. However, the principles apply to all surveys whether they are to describe disease or to provide valid patient perspectives.

- Surveys cost time and money. It is important to ensure that the information wanted is not available from routine sources.
- There should be a clear aim for the survey. What disease, or risk factor, is being measured? What is the case definition? What is the population of interest?
- Good planning is needed. Staff and resources will be needed to carry out the survey and produce a report.
- The sample size for the survey must be calculated. This is usually a balance between the need for precision (more precise estimates of incidence and prevalence require larger samples) and the resources and time available.
- Recruitment of the sample must be considered. A sampling frame must be chosen and from this the sample selected randomly, systematically or purposefully.
- The survey instrument (whether it be a symptom questionnaire, quality of life measure, physiological measurement, or laboratory test) should be valid, reliable, and repeatable.
- Steps should be taken to ensure a high response rate. Questionnaires should be piloted.

---

Criteria such as these may seem arbitrary but are, or at least should be, based on the probability of the future occurrence of specified outcomes known to be associated with the relevant condition. They may be based on the presence of physical signs or symptoms, or on physiological or biochemical characteristics which need to be measured by appropriate and standardised tests, for example valid and repeatable questionnaires, or physiological or biochemical tests. The criteria may change from time to time as further knowledge accrues but should not vary from place to place if estimates of incidence and prevalence are to be at all generalisable.

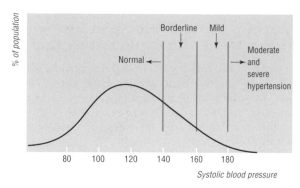

*Figure 2.2   Classification of hypertension by systolic blood pressure shows the continuum from normal to abnormal.*

## Incidence and prevalence

Incidence and prevalence are measures fundamental to the science of epidemiology. Both of these require the estimation of the *numerator* – the number of new cases observed (in the case of incidence) or the number of cases present in a population (in the case of prevalence) – and the estimation of the *denominator* – the number of people in the population "at risk". Incidence is a rate (that is, has a time dimension), prevalence is a proportion which is measured at a point in time but does not have a time dimension.

Neither prevalence nor incidence necessarily equate with need but knowledge of these parameters is usually an essential starting point for the assessment of need. Prevalence increases if incidence (or the rate of relapse) increases. It also increases if the rate of mortality (or remission) decreases. The relationship between these variables is best summarised as the "prevalence pool" concept (Figure 2.3).

Only a part of this prevalence pool may be visible at any one time if any proportion of the existing cases of a disease remains unrecognised. Unrecognised cases may be those at an early stage of development or may be the least severe, but neither of these is necessarily the case.

In health needs assessment it may be important to estimate both incidence and prevalence. The former is particularly important for diseases or conditions that are of short duration (for example, many communicable diseases) or for those for which a substantial amount of the health care input occurs shortly after diagnosis

15

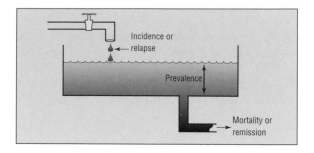

*Figure 2.3   Prevalence pool.*

(for example, myocardial infarction). Prevalence is particularly important when the duration of disease is long, for example, asthma, diabetes, or multiple sclerosis. Several types of incidence

---

### Box 2.2   Different types of incidence and prevalence

- "Stratum specific" estimates: "age specific" – for those in a given age group – for example
- "Crude" estimates: That is, crudely calculated by summing the numerator over all strata (for example, all ages) and dividing by the denominator of the total population
- "Standardised" estimates: that is, taking into account that the populations being compared may differ in terms of age or another important attribute

---

and prevalence may be used in needs assessment (see box above).

Standardised estimates may be derived by the "direct" or "indirect" methods. In the former, the stratum-specific estimates are taken from the population being standardised (this might be a town or locality) and applied to the stratum-specific population figures of the standard population (that of the country, for example); thus the incidence or prevalence, which would pertain in that population if those of the town or locality were applied to it, is calculated. In the latter, the process is reversed. The direct method is more usual and, in most cases, preferable. The main justifications for using the indirect rather than the direct method are:

- when the data items required for the indirect method are not available and
- when small numbers in the stratum-specific estimates in the population being standardised make them statistically unstable.

The Standardised Mortality Ratio (SMR) is a ratio derived from the technique of indirect standardisation.

## Generalisability

The NHS Management Executive set up the District Health Authority project in 1990 to support health authorities in their responsibility for assessing needs. This led to a series of health care needs assessment reviews.[3] The aim of these reviews was to give practical guidance to purchasers on moving from a service-led to a needs-led health care system. They provided an "off the shelf" guide to population needs for important health topics such as asthma and stroke.

However, information derived from elsewhere is often disregarded on the grounds that "it's not like that here". Standard epidemiological tools and guidance are extremely important. However, existing techniques are often crude, particularly when measuring morbidity. In the absence of dedicated research, evidence of morbidity is often derived from mortality data and, when research is available, extrapolation to different populations can disguise underlying variations.[6] Clearly, populations will differ in age, gender, socioeconomic or ethnic mix, or other attributes, or they may be other legitimate reasons for thinking that work carried out elsewhere is not applicable (use of an incorrect case definition, for example). Issues of generalisability can usually be divided into four broad areas:

- Case definitions: are they acceptable?
- The time since the study was carried out: is the information still timely?
- Is the study sound in other respects, (for example, methods of ascertainment (numerators) and demographic information (denominators), and
- Have the data been presented (or are they available) for the relevant strata of known confounders?

17

The term "confounders" is used here to encompass attributes which influence incidence and/or prevalence such as age, gender, and socioeconomic or ethnic group.

Diabetes is an example of a condition for which knowledge of incidence and prevalence in relation to confounders is essential if any valid estimate of need is to be made. In general practices which are known to have identified their diabetic patients comprehensively, diabetes prevalence shows a close and totally expected relationship with the proportion of the practice list aged 65 years and over.[7] Thus, for practices who are unsure of the completeness of their diabetes registers, some indication of how close they are to complete ascertainment can be derived by comparing their observed prevalence figure with that expected on the basis of this relationship with age. However, this only holds if the practice population has a similar composition, in terms of ethnic origin, to the practices on which the initial observations have been made. Since it is known that the prevalence of diabetes varies between ethnic groups and, equally important, that the relationship between prevalence and age is different in different ethnic groups, the effect on prevalence of the ethnic composition of the practice needs to be taken into account.

Although no convincing relationship has been demonstrated between diabetes prevalence and socioeconomic group, relationships have been demonstrated between diabetes outcomes and socioeconomic status with, as would be expected, worse outcomes in the more disadvantaged groups. For this reason, any estimate of need ("the ability to benefit from care"[1]) for diabetes services must take socioeconomic status into account.

If the four aspects described above are satisfied then there is no reason why information from other localities cannot be applied to the local situation. To do so, with all reasonable care, can save precious resources which might otherwise be squandered in carrying out yet another health needs assessment on a given health problem merely because of a misplaced enthusiasm for locally derived data.

"Locality based health needs assessment" (that is, needs assessment dealing with populations smaller than district health authorities or their equivalents) has the advantage of allowing knowledge of the local scene to be used in the planning of local services. As argued above, the use of local data, to the exclusion of data available from elsewhere, needs to be carefully considered. Apart from the cost implications of repeating locally what may have been done perfectly well elsewhere and can be extrapolated, there are statistical considerations that need to be taken into account when the frequency of relatively rare events is assessed. Even diseases that are common enough to be regarded as major public health problems (for example, carcinoma of the cervix), occur relatively infrequently in small populations.

Three important issues need to be taken into account when deciding the minimum size of the population on which a needs assessment should be based. These are:

(1) the frequency of occurrence (incidence, prevalence or both);
(2) the impact that the condition makes on those who suffer from it, and
(3) the cost implications of treatment.

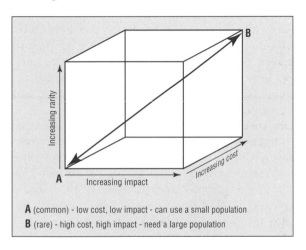

A (common) - low cost, low impact - can use a small population
B (rare) - high cost, high impact - need a large population

*Figure 2.4   Attributes of a health problem to consider when deciding the size of the population for a needs assessment.*

For a rare condition with a high impact on sufferers and carers and with high treatment costs (for example, childhood leukaemia), a relatively large population needs to be studied for a worthwhile needs assessment. The extent of need for common, low impact, low cost conditions can be assessed on smaller populations. For a single practice it would be unwise to base the assessment of need for conditions with a prevalence of less than 1%. So whereas a needs assessment for childhood leukaemia would be of limited value for a population much less than 1 million, a needs assessment for mild depression could be based on the population served by an average four-doctor practice.

The NHS, in common with many other organisations, devotes more care and resource to collecting data than it does to using the data it collects. Routine sources of information are not as comprehensive as in some countries (for example, the Scandinavian countries) but they do exist, and it is surprising

---

## Box 2.3 National sources of health information in the United Kingdom

- *Population*: Census data can be used to describe populations at a district or electoral ward level by age, gender, ethnicity, or socioeconomic status. Census information on variables such as unemployment and overcrowding can be used to produce indices of deprivation for electoral wards, for example the Jarman Index and Townsend Score.
- *Mortality*: National registration of deaths and causes of death provide comprehensive (though not always accurate) mortality information. Perinatal and infant mortality "rates" (they are not rates but proportions) are used for comparisons of the quality of health care. Standardised Mortality Rates are used to compare local information on total mortality or mortality from specific causes.
- *Morbidity*: National and local registers provide data of variable accuracy. Registers exist for: cancers (type of cancer, treatment, and survival); drug addiction; congenital abnormalities; specific diseases (such as diabetes and stroke). Communicable disease notification provides a source of information for local surveillance. The RCGP Unit collects morbidity data from sample practices around the UK. Prescribing data can be a valuable surrogate marker of morbidity. Insurance companies can be an important source of health information in countries with largely insurance-based systems.
- *Health care*: Hospital activity data can provide information on hospital admissions, diagnoses, length of stay, operations performed, and patient characteristics. Clinical indicators such as the Health Service Indicators can provide information on the comparative performance of hospitals and health authorities.

---

how infrequently they are used or even known about (see box below).

Unfortunately, "Murphy's Law of Information" plays a part at this stage: "The information we have is not what we want. The information we want is not what we need. The information we need is too expensive to collect." Despite that pessimistic view, it is possible to make use of routinely available data even if this entails some compromise in terms of precision. The next box illustrates how routinely collected data can be used with survey information to provide a powerful assessment of health needs and use of services.

---

## Box 2.4  Example of an epidemiological health needs assessment[8]

- *Objective:* To assess whether the use of health services by people with coronary heart disease reflected need.
- *Setting:* Health authority with a population of 530 000.
- *Methods:* The prevalence of angina was determined by a validated postal questionnaire. Routine health data were collected on SMRs; admission rates for coronary heart disease and operation rates for angiography, angioplasty, and coronary heart disease. Census data were used to calculate Townsend scores to describe deprivation for electoral wards. Prevalence of angina and use of services were then compared with deprivation scores for each ward.
- *Results:* Angina and mortality from heart disease were more common in wards with high deprivation scores. However, treatment by revascularisation procedures was more common in more affluent wards.
- *Conclusion:* The use of revascularisation services was not commensurate with need. Steps should be taken to ensure health care is targeted to those who most need it.

---

# References

1 Stevens A, Raftery J. Introduction. In: Stevens A, Raftery J, eds. *Health care needs assessment*. Oxford: Radcliffe Medical Press Ltd, Vol 1, 1994.
2 Last JM. *A dictionary of epidemiology*. 3rd edn. Oxford: Oxford University Press, 1995.

---

## Summary points

- Epidemiological methods can be used to describe health needs in terms of the distribution of specific diseases.

- Although incidence and prevalence do not necessarily equate with need, they are both important in describing the population burden of disease.

- Specific epidemiological studies can be expensive and time consuming. Existing information from previous studies can be used to inform local needs if criteria for generalisability are met.

- Routine sources of health information can suffer from inaccuracy and inappropriateness. However, they can provide valuable descriptions of health and health care use in a defined population.

---

3 Subcommittee of WHO/ISH Mild Hypertension Liaison Committee. Summary of 1993 World Health Organisation – International Society of Hypertension guidelines for the management of mild hypertension. *BMJ* 1993;307:1541–6.

4 National Asthma Education Program: Expert Panel Report. *Guidelines for the diagnosis and management of asthma.* Bethesda: US Department of Health and Human Services, 1991.

5 World Health Organisation Study Group. *Diabetes mellitus.* Technical Report Series No. 727. Geneva: World Health Organisation, 1985.

6 Doyal L. Needs, rights and equity: moral quality in healthcare rationing. *Quality in Health Care* 1995;4:273–83.

7 Williams R. Diabetes. In: Stevens A, Raftery J, eds. *Health Care Needs Assessment.* Oxford: Radcliffe Medical Press Ltd, Vol 1, 1994.

8 Payne N, Saul C. Variations in use of cardiology services in a health authority: comparison of coronary artery revascularisation rates with prevalence of angina and coronary mortality. *BMJ* 1997;314:257–61.

# 3 The development of practical approaches to health needs assessment

ANDREW STEVENS and STEPHEN GILLAM

The purpose of this chapter is to link the theory and practice of health care needs assessment. Having set out key theoretical elements we consider the practical approaches used and the challenges they present.

The *purpose* of needs assessment in health care is to gather the information required to bring about change beneficial to the health of the population. It is generally, but not universally, accepted that this takes place within the context of finite resources.[1] "Health gain" can therefore be achieved by reallocating resources as a result of identifying:

- non-recipients of beneficial health care interventions (that is, unmet need);
- recipients of ineffective health care (and releasing the resources for unmet need);
- recipients of inefficient health care (and releasing resources for unmet need), and
- recipients of inappropriate health care (for whom the outcomes could be improved).

The *subjects* of health care needs assessment are the populations and patients who are health care recipients or potential beneficiaries of health care. Populations, of course, include individual patients. The assessment of individuals' needs may form part of the assessment of a population's needs, but may be costly and risks ignoring unseen individuals. The circumstances favouring individual needs assessment for planning purposes are set out in Table 3.1.

Table 3.1   When to assess health care needs on an individual and population basis

| Parameter | Individual | Population |
|-----------|-----------|-----------|
| Case-load | Few | Many |
| Cost per patient | High | Low |
| Hidden patients | Few | Many |
| Case-mix variability | High | Low |

The priority attached to different needs, whether population or individual raises philosophical problems. For example, should the principal criterion be the benefit that could potentially be obtained for each individual, or the severity of their presenting condition?[2] In other words should greater priority (that is, a greater assessed need) be attributed to an early stage colorectal cancer patient's need for surgery or to a terminally ill lung cancer patient's need for hospice care? In practice the former, the approach that favours the greater benefit, takes precedence in formal needs assessment, but not exclusively. In either case cost always enters the equation. There are some marginal benefits that cannot be afforded in a publicly funded system because of the other treatments and benefits that need to be sacrificed to fund them.

New *practitioners* of needs assessment are emerging. The *New NHS* white paper requires primary care groups to contribute to health authorities' health improvement programmes "helping to ensure that they reflect the perspectives of the local community and the experiences of local patients". More GPs will therefore face the dilemmas that needs assessment is intended to tackle.

## From theory to practice

Different frameworks for health care needs assessment have reflected different purposes as well as different times and contexts.[4] The life-cycle model, for example, is a framework which encourages needs assessors to think comprehensively about different population groups according to age.[5] It is an attractive model because of its simplicity, but does not distinguish need and demand, or emphasise the pivotal theme of "capacity to benefit".

A particular purpose of health care needs assessment is the spatial allocation of resources. Geographical equity between regions, districts, and even localities (for example, housing estates), can be addressed by global and surrogate measures of health, particularly deprivation indices and standardised mortality ratios.[6] Measuring relative deprivation is a step forward from approaches which do not distinguish need from supply and demand, but it cannot be used to specify precise needs in a service planning sense. In short, measuring deprivation tells us whether Burnley is less well resourced than Belgravia, but does not help in deciding the number of coronary care beds needed in either.

The definition of "need as the capacity to benefit" represents a further advance because it can be directed at specific services.[7-9] It has generated new practical approaches in an area of sometimes paralysing controversy. The following points apply to needs assessment undertaken both at the level of health authority and general practice:

- The *population's ability to benefit* from health care equals the aggregate of individuals' ability to benefit. For most health problems (but see Table 3.1) this will be more readily deducible from epidemiological data than from clinical records.
- The *ability to benefit* does not mean that every outcome will be favourable, but rather that need implies potential benefit, which on average is effective.
- The *benefit* is not just a change in clinical status, but can include reassurance, supportive care and the relief of carers. The list of beneficiaries of care can extend beyond the patient to families and carers.
- *Health care* includes not just treatment, but also prevention, diagnosis, continuing care, rehabilitation, and palliative care.[8]

We argue that such benefits are ideally assessed by a mixed epidemiological and cost effectiveness approach, supplemented by "corporate" and "comparative" methods.[8,9] All of these methods include the enumeration of current services, but there are a variety of other contemporary approaches to service-related needs assessment which should be noted. These include not just population health care needs assessment but also social services assessments, individual health care needs assessment, participatory and Oregon-style planning, population and client group surveys, expert speciality recommendations, and clinical effectiveness research.[10] Their usefulness can be assessed using the following criteria:

(1) Is the needs assessment about populations or individuals?

(2) Is there a clear context of allocating scarce resources (that is, are the needs assessed in the context of priority setting among competing needs)?

(3) Is the needs assessment exploratory or definitive (that is, is the object to clarify what should be done, or just to highlight problems which are accompanied by no obvious intervention)?

(4) Is the determination of the most important needs based on expert knowledge or participatory methods?

Table 3.2 shows how other approaches compare with population health care needs assessment based on the capacity to benefit. In population health care needs assessment the concern is with the health of populations with a common condition or presentation – for example, all patients with diabetes (known or not known) on a practice list. It recognises that resources are finite and avoids focusing on advocacy for individual groups without considering competing priorities. It is definitive rather than exploratory in that client groups are considered together with actual interventions; by contrast, this is not a feature of some lifestyle or disability surveys; for example, the needs are determined by expert appraisal of the evidence rather than principally through public participation. However, any approach which contributes information on *numbers* in a particular group, that is, incidence and prevalence, the *effectiveness* and cost effectiveness of interventions, and the distribution of *current services* and their costs will be useful in practice.

## Defining base-line services

Measured needs only takes on meaning in relation to the existing services. Needs assessment is about change and it is essential to know what to change from as well as what to change to. Several steps are involved. First, the service under consideration has to be disaggregated into meaningful subunits. For example, mental health can be split up into adult, elderly, child, forensic, substance abuse, etc. Adult mental health, could then be further subdivided as services for long stay, short stay, day care, community treatment, and so forth. Each of these encompasses a variety of different interventions. There follows a decision on what to measure. Structural factors such as bed capacity, staffing levels, and costs

Table 3.2  Different approaches to health care needs assessment

| Criterion | Individual/population-based | Resource scarcity clear | Definitive/explanatory | Expert/participatory |
|---|---|---|---|---|
| Population health care needs | Population | Yes | Definitive | Expert |
| Individual health care needs | Individual | Sometimes | Definitive | Expert |
| Social services assessments | Individual | Sometimes | Both | Both |
| Participatory planning | Population | Sometimes | Definitive | Participatory |
| Oregon-style planning | Population | Yes | Definitive | Both |
| Population surveys | Population | No | Exploratory | Expert |
| Client group surveys | Population | No | Exploratory | Both |
| Speciality recommendations | Population | No | Definitive | Expert |
| Effectiveness reviews | Population | Yes | Definitive | Expert |

(Adapted with permission from *Health care needs assessment* (eds A Stevens, J Raftery), Oxford: Radcliffe Medical Press, 1997.)

provide a powerful starting point. Measurement of process (for example, throughput) and outcomes (for example, death rate) will have little meaning unless case mix and severity are well defined. A plausible mental health base-line service specification focusing on structure and cost is set out in Table 3.3. The emphasis is on obtaining the key information needed to summarise existing levels of service as succinctly as possible.[11]

Table 3.3  Example of a table of base-line services

| Resource name | Resource function | Capacity | Unit cost | Notes on quality/ performance |
|---|---|---|---|---|
| Acute ward A | Acute assessment | Beds | £1000 per bed | Nurse morale problems |
| Community team B | Community support for mild/stable conditions | Places | £1000 per place | Poor coordination with general practice |
| Long-stay facility C | Long-stay/ dementia | Beds | £1000 per bed | Being run down |

(Adapted with permission from *Measuring mental health needs* (eds G Thornicroft, C Brewin, J Wing), London: Gaskell, 1992.)

## Corporate approaches

The "corporate approach" involves the systematic collection of the knowledge and views of informants on health care services and needs. Valuable information is often available from health authority staff, provider clinicians, and general practitioners, as well as from users. Figure 3.1 lists possible informants. While such an approach blurs the distinction between need and demand, and between science and vested interest, the intimate, detailed knowledge of interested parties amassed over years might otherwise be overlooked. Furthermore, the corporate approach is essential if policies are to be sensitive to local circumstances. Eliciting local views is not the same as being bound by them. It allows sensitivity to local circumstances, particularly those consequent on historical provision. The unmet needs of discharged seriously mentally ill people from closed long-stay hospitals, or the absence of primary care for homeless groups may only be readily uncovered by speaking to people. Where cost effectiveness considerations are otherwise equal, local concerns may justifiably attach priorities to particular

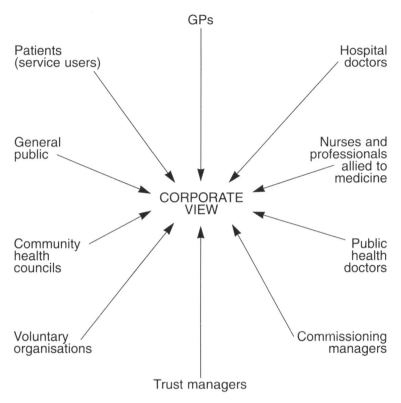

*Figure 3.1   Corporate informants (adapted with permission from Stevens A, Raftery J, eds.* Health care needs assessment, the epidemiologically based needs assessment reviews. *Oxford: Radcliffe Medical Press, Vol. 1, 1994.)*

services. Furthermore, local experience and involvement will make any needs assessment easier to defend.

## Comparative approaches

The "comparative approach" to needs assessment contrasts the services received by the population in one area with those received elsewhere. If nothing else is known about the optimum service to be provided, there is at least reason for investigation if the level of service differs markedly from that provided elsewhere. Comparisons have proved very powerful tools for investigating health services.[12,13] For example, the need to raise renal dialysis and transplantation levels from 20 per million in the 1960s to 80 per million was suggested by comparison with European countries and subsequently confirmed epidemiologically.[14] New performance indicator packages are being piloted in both primary and secondary care.[15] While they require sensitive interpretation, comparative process and outcome indicators may help identify deficiencies in service provision.

## Epidemiological/cost effectiveness approaches

The essence of needs assessment is an understanding of what is effective and for whom. Critical steps involve:

(1) A clear statement of the population group whose needs are to be assessed (normally a group who share the same pathology). In the case of a needs assessment for diabetic services, this might include both known and latent diabetics. In the case of substance misuse it would include past, present, and potential misusers.

(2) Identifying subcategories of this population (perhaps "health benefit groups") with particular service needs. People with type 1 (insulin dependent) diabetes would be distinguished from Those with type 2 (non-insulin dependent) diabetes. Current dependent substance misusers would be distinguished from intoxicated misusers, those with comorbidities, those in recovery (at risk of relapse), and those at risk of becoming new users.

(3) Setting out the prevalence and incidence of the subcategories. How many of each are there?

(4) Setting out the current services available (the baseline discussed above) – all services whether in primary, secondary care, or elsewhere.

(5) Identifying the effectiveness and cost effectiveness of interventions and services associated – the essence of evidence based health care.

(6) Setting out a model of care which apportions relative priorities.[9,10]

As a general rule, establishing the effectiveness of an intervention must be the most important step. There is little point in counting potential beneficiaries for an intervention which is of no benefit. Most challenging of all is the task of apportioning relative priority to different services and recipients. Cost effectiveness must be taken into consideration. The use of unitary cost-utility measures can be helpful where available, and decision matrices render decision making more explicit. However, flexibility around particular patient circumstances is often required.

## Managing the task

Several challenges are commonly encountered in understanding needs assessment. Firstly the mosaic of information required for needs assessment reflects its key components, that is, establishing existing services, prevalence, and incidence of client groups (subcategorised appropriately), and the effectiveness of interventions. The evidence based medicine movement has made access to information – from hand searching through electronic databases to evidence based compendia – progressively easier in the effectiveness field.[16,17] The same cannot be said of information available on epidemiology or services provided. Good quality local data on health service structure and utilisation can be surprisingly difficult to obtain. The absence of common disease definitions, common classification systems and compatible software, and the partial recording of activity, limits the value of many databases.[18]

The triangulation of information sources is therefore critical. Useful information can be either local or national, either numerical or textual, and collected either routinely or *ad hoc*. Figure 3.2 sets out a number of key intelligence items for the needs assessors.[19] The task is greatly facilitated with the help of a skilled librarian with access to a basic range of texts and databases. National sources of both epidemiological and effectiveness data offer health care needs assessors a firm starting point for their work.

A second challenge is the involvement of health professionals in health care needs assessment. The traditionally individualistic approach of doctors in particular may be difficult to reconcile with the utilitarian approach of planners with a population focus. The latter implies a fundamental reappraisal of the doctor's role and the balance of power within the doctor/patient relationship.[20] It is also important not to neglect the contribution of other health professionals. For example, in primary care much information is collected by community nursing staff, and health visitors' skills, in particular, are easily overlooked.[21] Even where doctors and nurses

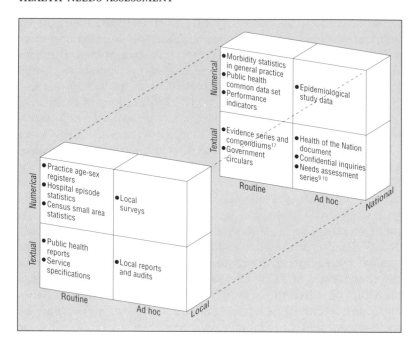

*Figure 3.2   Intelligence sources: examples.*

have a population focus, needs assessment has opportunity costs; not everyone can devote time to it, but at the very least, ensuring target efficiency, that is ensuring that services are directed first to the individuals with the greatest potential benefit, is a key clinical task.

Thirdly, needs assessment is futile if it does not result in improved services to patients. A key to successful needs assessment is the proper understanding of its relationship to the rest of the planning process. Too much needs assessment is divorced from managers' deadlines and priorities. If the information and recommendations produced are not timely, they will not be useful. The results of needs assessment therefore need to be encapsulated in strategies or business plans. These need clear definitions of objectives, describing what needs to be done, by whom, and by when.[22] The key to effecting change is an understanding of the opportunities that may facilitate and the obstacles that may obstruct what is being attempted – knowing which "levers" to use. An understanding of the sources of finance, their planning cycles, and the criteria used to fund new initiatives is essential. Health authorities/boards clearly indicate the timing of development bids and the structure of applications that they wish to be submitted.

A fourth challenge is to ensure that needs assessment is not just effective but efficient and cost effective. Little is known of the cost effectiveness of needs assessment. But at least one survey found it to be effective in leading to service change at little cost.[23] Evaluation of different purchasing models should help to clarify the population sizes for which needs assessment for different services is most efficiently undertaken.[24]

## Conclusion

In practice, although needs assessment represents an amalgam of epidemiology, economics, and values, it has to be turned into a practical tool, but the reification of needs assessment has two unfortunate effects. Firstly, it is unhelpful to see the outcome of needs assessment as a document – the culmination of a series of easily defined, finite steps. Rather needs assessment is an iterative, sometimes messy, process that may serve a number of different political purposes. The most important of these is to develop a consensus among planners, managers, and clinicians regarding service development priorities. Secondly, needs assessment is too easily seen as some arcane preserve of public health specialists. The technical skills required can be exaggerated.[25] Basic numeracy and commonsense are the most important prerequisites.

The current approaches to needs assessment may turn out to be time and context limited. Much needs assessment activity was stimulated by the advent of an internal market and by doubts about the cost effectiveness and appropriateness of care. Health authorities and GPs in their role as purchasers require detailed service specification for the first time. However, with increasing evidence for the equivocal efficacy of many health care interventions, of delayed uptake of effective health care,[26] unexplained geographical variations, and of rising costs, the concern with capacity to benefit within finite resources is unlikely to wane. The rhetoric may therefore change but the demand for increasingly sophisticated approaches to needs assessment will intensify.

---

**Summary points**

- Health care need is the capacity to benefit from health care.
- The assessment of population benefit includes a measure of epidemiology (how many) and cost effectiveness (how good).
- Other sources, especially comparisons and corporate knowledge, can contribute usefully.
- An optimal approach requires a good intelligence facility, clinical involvement and a close relation to the planning process.

---

# References

1 Dixon, J, Harrison A, New B. Is the NHS underfunded? *BMJ* 1997;**314**:58–61.
2 Culyer A. Need: the idea won't do – but we still need it. *Soc Sci Med* 1955;**40**: 727–30.
3 Department of Health. *The new NHS, modern, dependable.* London: HMSO, 1997.
4 Stevens A, Gabbay J. Needs assessment, needs assessment. *Health trends* 1991; **23**:20–3
5 Pickin C. *Assessment of health need using the life cycle framework.* Manchester: Northwestern RHA, 1991.
6 Department of Health and Social Security. *Sharing resources for health in England.* Report of the Resource Allocation Working Party. London: DHSS, 1976.
7 Culyer A. *Need and the National Health Service.* London: Martin Robertson, 1976.
8 National Health Service Management Executive. *Assessing health care needs.* London: Department of Health, 1991.
9 Stevens A, Raftery J. Introduction. In: Stevens A, Raftery J, eds. *Health care needs assessment, the epidemiologically based needs assessment reviews.* Oxford: Radcliffe Medical Press, Vol. 1, 1994.
10 Stevens A, Raftery J. Introduction: Alternative approaches to health care needs assessment. In: Stevens A, Raftery J, eds. *Health care needs assessment.* Second Series. Oxford: Radcliffe Medical Press, 1997.
11 Stevens A, Raftery J. The purchasers' information requirements on mental health needs and contracting for mental health services. In: Thornicroft G, Brewin C, Wing J, eds. *Measuring mental health needs.* London: Gaskell, 1992.
12 Saunders D, Coulter A, McPherson K. *Varieties in hospital admission rates; a review of the literature.* London: King's Fund, 1989.
13 Wennberg JE, Malley AG, Hanley D, *et al.* An assessment of prostatectomy for benign urinary tract obstruction. Geographic variations and the evaluation of medical care outcomes. *J Am Med Assoc* 1988;**259**:3027–30.
14 Beech R, Gulliford M, Mays N, *et al.* Renal disease. In: Stevens A, Raftery J, eds. *Health care needs assessment, the epidemiologically based needs assessment reviews.* Oxford: Radcliffe Medical Press, Vol. 1, 1994.
15 NHS Executive. *Consulting the NHS on a set of provisional clinical indicators.* EL(97)49. Leeds: NHSE, 1997.
16 Haynes B, Sackett D, Muir Gray J, Cook D, Guyatt C. Transferring evidence from research into practice: 2: Getting the evidence straight. *Evidence Based Medicine* 1997,**2**:4–6.

17 Booth A. *Scharr guide to evidence based practice.* University of Sheffield: Scharr Occasional Paper no. 97/2. Sheffield School of health and related research, 1997.
18 Pringle M, Hobbs R. Large computer databases in general practice. *BMJ* 1991; **302**:742–3
19 NHS Management Executive. *Purchasing intelligence.* London: Department of Health, 1991.
20 Gillam S, Murray A. *Needs assessment in general practice.* London: Royal College of General Practitioners, Occasional Paper No 73, 1996.
21 Royal College of Nursing. *The GP practice population profiles. A framework for every member of the primary health care team.* London: RCN, 1993.
22 Spiegel N, Murphy E, Kinmonth AL *et al.* Managing change in general practice: a step by step guide. *BMJ* 1992;**304**:231–4.
23 Fulop N, Henscher M. *A survey of needs assessment activity in London health authorities.* London: Kings Fund, 1997.
24 Mays N, Goodwin, Bevan G, Wike S (on behalf of TP-net). *Total purchasing: a profile of national pilot projects.* London: Kings Fund, 1997.
25 Gillam SJ. Assessing populations' health needs: the general practitioners' contribution. *Br J Gen Pract* 1992;**42**:404.
26 Antman E, Lau J, Kupelnick B, Mosteller F, Chalmers T. A comparison of results of meta-analyses of randomised control trials and recommendations of experts. *J Am Med Ass* 1992;**268**:240–48.

# 4 Needs assessment in primary care – I

JOHN WILKINSON and SCOTT A MURRAY

## The central role of primary care

In the United Kingdom, general practitioners have a central role in determining who receives hospital care. General practitioners assess their patients' needs daily for both primary and secondary care. With very few exceptions, in order for patients to be seen in a hospital, they must be referred by a general practitioner. This can avoid unnecessary referrals and can also ensure that a generalist is involved in the patient at an early stage.

The needs of patients are a central element of the new NHS white papers.[1,2] Until now, general practitioners have had patchy involvement in the commissioning of health care. This role is now to be strengthened by the creation of primary care groups. This will also lead to more involvement of the local community and other professionals – such as community nurses and social service departments of the local authority. General practitioners as commissioners of primary care groups will in future be able to determine much more directly how and where health care is provided for their patients. General practitioners are also centrally placed to have a wider influence on health within their community.

General practitioners have traditionally based their referral decisions (and hence purchasing) for health care on their own judgement and experience, whereas health authority purchasers have increasingly attempted to base decisions on systematic, epidemiologically informed assessments of need. No one really knows which is the more effective technique, but it may be that there are lessons to be learnt from a combined approach which also includes a more systematic method of "judgement".[3] Here we examine ways in which these two approaches can be combined.

## Influence on needs and demands

Primary health care teams are adept at identifying individual patients' needs. Health needs assessment is generally taken to mean the consideration of the whole practice's needs or a subset of the population within the practice. This subset may be a group of patients with special needs such as single mothers or may relate to a geographical community or a disease-based group.

The relationship between needs demand and supply was described in Chapter 1 and is no less applicable in the primary care setting. In short a "health need" implies that the practice population or groups within it would benefit from a particular health intervention. The box illustrates an example of this.

---

### Box 4.1   Need, demand, and supply for the treatment of sore throats

- *Demand* Patients often expect and demand treatment for a sore throat with antibiotics.
- *Supply* Antibiotics are available for the treatment of sore throats and often doctors are willing to prescribe.
- *Need* Antibiotics have a limited role in the management of sore throats, most being viral in origin.[4]

---

### Box 4.2   Major influences on needs, demand and supply

- *Demand* (what people ask for): patients, politicians, pressure groups, media.
- *Supply* (what is provided): health professionals, trust managers, health authorities, primary health care teams.
- *Need* (what people might benefit from): health authority, public health physicians, health planners.

---

The second box illustrates where some of the main influences of demand, supply, and need have traditionally been found. Over the past few years, little attention has been paid to meeting the needs of patients. Demand and supply issues have been the main focus of attention, with, for example the management of waiting lists having a high political profile. Waiting lists are more closely related to demand and supply than to need. Traditional assessors of needs such as public health physicians have focused their activities largely elsewhere and only recently has the language of planning returned in place of the rhetoric of market forces. There is a need to involve all these individuals and groups more closely in needs assessment rather than to leave this important work solely to health planners and public health physicians.

## Do we get involved with wider health needs?

Health professionals understandably tend to think of health needs in terms of services that they can provide, whereas patients may have different ideas about what affects their health. This might include getting a job, having a roof over their head, having a bus route which makes getting to see the doctor easy. A practice may decide that they do not have the time and resources to consider these types of needs and feel even less confident about being able to do anything about such needs, but if primary care has the aim of improving the health status of individuals as well as providing health services, such factors must at least be identified for action by someone else. Lalonde[5] when Minister of Health in Canada emphasised the importance of lifestyles and the environment on health as well as the influences of human biology and health care provision. A practice may alternatively decide to look at a particular issue facing some of their patients, for example the needs of patients with diabetes,[6] but even such focused needs assessments should involve patients in the process.

## Levels for needs assessment

Needs can be assessed at various levels, from international, national, regional, locality, groups of practices, practices, small geographic neighbourhoods, and individual level.

- *International.* Needs assessment at this level may be undertaken by the World Health Organisation, the European Union, or international aid agencies
- *National.* The current NHS national priorities are cancer and mental health. Practices may decide that they wish to work collaboratively with their local health authority/board on assessing needs, for example for cancer services: it might be a high priority to examine the needs of patients requiring palliative care locally. The advantage of tackling some national priorities is that it may be easier to persuade health authorities/boards to fund identified gaps in services. The most common complaints presented by patients – stress, arthritis, and dyspepsia – have never been identified as national priorities.[7]
- *Regional.* Some priorities may be identified on a subnational level, perhaps at county level. The need for a liver transplantation service could be assessed at this level.
- *Health authority/board.* The needs for neonatal care, obstetric care, or dietetics are sometimes assessed at this level.
- *Locality.* The creation of primary care groups will lead to increasing importance for needs assessment to be undertaken at this level. It may be appropriate for some more common conditions or where there is a single provider of services for practices to combine to undertake needs assessment. Generally larger populations will produce more robust results. There is also no need for every practice to carry out similar types of needs assessment when it is unlikely that there will be different needs between practices. Issues suitable for tackling at this level might include unwanted pregnancy, dental caries, inequalities in service provision of community nursing.
- *Practice specific.* It is worth thinking about a single piece of needs assessment work where a practice is relatively large and is situated in an area of particular need. Single practice approaches seem to work best when there is underlying disadvantage, and the practice may wish to consider the wider influences on the health of their population. Issues such as mental health and drug addiction may be particularly relevant to an individual practice.
- *Small neighbourhood.* Some practices have a group of patients who live in a well defined disadvantaged area. Such a group can usefully be engaged in a needs assessment exercise and brought into the planning process.

- *Individual level.* This is frequently performed daily in consultations by general practitioners and nurses.

## Who to involve

A practical example of how involvement at many levels led to change is given in the box below.

---

### Box 4.3   Practical example of how needs assessment can lead to changes

An area surrounding the army garrison in Catterick, North Yorkshire was identified as an area of special need. A multiagency approach (involving local GPs, parish council, social services, health authority and health promotion, local business) was developed which involved rapid participatory appraisal and local surveys. Initially this led to the health authority appointing a community development worker. Since that time a number of significant developments have occurred in the area. The local practice premises are to be rebuilt. A chemist and a dentist have set up premises in the area. The local college has established a base. A partnership with local business has been set up which submitted a successful bid of £1.5 million for the Government's Special Regeneration Bid (SRB) aimed at improving the economic infrastructure in the area as well as providing local facilities for sport and fitness.

---

### Involve all members of the practice team

The general practitioner, armed with personal knowledge from individual consultations, home visits, and key facts and figures concerning his practice population is ideally placed to assess local health needs, but health needs assessment must not be viewed as an activity for the doctors alone Other members of the primary health care team possess information that can provide valuable insights into the needs of the practice population. Health visitors have information on preschool children, and indeed have a specific public health role.[8] Many health visitors undertake practice profiling that can be of direct benefit to the practice, whilst district nurses daily visit the elderly and housebound. Soft intelligence (for example, from local newspapers, local pressure groups) may be of equal value, particularly in identifying areas in which further needs assessment work is required. The practice manager and receptionists may understand global health problems in the community or those which affect groupings within the practice. It is important to consider involving all staff in the practice at an early stage in health needs assessment.

### Involve the public

Any practice or group of practices needs to decide how the public will be involved at an early stage. Methods for involving the public have been described by May *et al.*[9]

### Involve the trusts and other providers of services

Those who provide care in primary, secondary, and tertiary care settings have an important role to play in health needs assessment. Consultants working in hospital or community trusts usually have a clear picture of the needs for their particular service. This can be a rich source of help and advice for general practitioners wishing to undertake needs assessment. Combining specialist expertise and the wide experience from general practice can produce valuable information. Hospital and community trusts themselves are a useful source of data for a practice. Other service providers should also be considered such as hospices and other agencies both in the statutory and voluntary sector.

### Informing local commissioning

Following the publication of the white paper on the future of the NHS, we now know that general practitioners, working closely with others, will be central to the commissioning of local services. The government intends to establish primary care groups which will bring together GPs and community nurses. Primary care groups will evolve from the wide range of local commissioning arrangements currently in place, supported by the health authority. These groups will take on a wide range of responsibilities depending on their stage of development. These responsibilities will range from an advisory role to the health authority to the creation of freestanding primary care trusts. These groups will typically serve populations of around 100000. The involvement of local community representatives and social services will greatly facilitate a multiagency approach to health needs assessment.

## Obstacles to undertaking health needs assessment in primary care[10]

In primary care anyone attempting needs assessment is likely to encounter some specific obstacles. Some of these are summarised below:

- *Ethical.* General practitioners are used to caring for individuals and families. Assessing and prioritising the needs of groups is less familiar territory for most GPs.
- *Skills shortage.* The skills to examine data and undertake surveys are relatively rare in general practice.
- *Lack of incentives.* There is a clear need for resources for general practitioners to undertake these type of activities.
- *Methodological.* There is no widely accepted approach to needs assessment in primary care.
- *Compartmentalisation.* Assessment of health needs may be seen as the responsibility of others.
- *Conflicting priorities.* These may be between addressing the local needs of the population and the needs set by national priorities.
- *Isolation.* Locality groups may provide the best forum for needs assessment in the future.
- *Relevance of the information.* Much of the information available at local level does not relate well to a general practice population.
- *Rationing.* May identifying needs lead to increased demand? It has been suggested that giving the population greater information does not necessarily lead to greater demands.[11]
- *Lack of evidence.* There is a dearth of evidence on effective methods of health needs assessment (especially in primary care).
- *Organisational uncertainty.* Organisational change is a constant feature of today's NHS; therefore short-term perspectives are commonplace (though the new white paper gives considerable emphasis to the role of needs assessment).
- *Accountability.* General practitioners are likely to find themselves increasingly accountable for the decisions they take involving the spending of public money.
- *Conceptual.* The conflict between the role of the patient advocate and responsibility for the local population.

- *Time*. Time is the biggest obstacle in busy general practice.
- *Support*. Most practices will need help and support in order to undertake effective needs assessment.
- *Quality of routine clinical data*. Routine clinical data from hospitals have been shown to contain many inaccuracies,[12] although it is known that the quality of some clinical databases has substantially improved in recent years.[13]
- *Assessing the information and interpreting the results*. Drawing conclusions from disparate range of information may be difficult (for example, referral rates, prescribing data).

## Hard-to-reach groups

### Assessing the needs

Concentrating needs assessment activity at a local level based primarily around general practice, may lead to the needs of certain groups being overlooked.[14] Primary care teams or locality groups therefore need to consider whether any important groups in their areas are being missed. The groups that merit special attention are listed in the box below.

---

**Box 4.4   Hard-to-reach groups**

- Ethnic and cultural minorities
- Travellers
- Refugees
- The homeless
- Sex workers
- Adolescents
- Rural communities.[16,17]

---

Localities may need to think whether there are any other groups with particular needs that may be hard to identify. For traditional practice-based approaches, patients need to be registered with a general practitioner. Primary care may not be readily accessible to high-risk groups for various reasons:

- *Patients failing to register*. Patients may not register for a variety of reasons. Some people will not seek to register with a doctor until they require medical help. This will be the case particularly

43

in age groups with good health, and will be the case with young single men. Some people will assume a link with the authorities and therefore illegal immigrants, substance abusers, and sex workers may fear that information may be passed onto the police. Some people may not understand the system or have had a bad experience when trying to register.

- *Reasons for not taking up services.* Patients may not take up services for a variety of reasons. These may include difficulties with the language or culture. Patients may have a different set of values; for example, the philosophy of altering behaviour today, such as stopping smoking, for a longer term benefit may not be an attractive proposition to a young mother who does not know how she is going to feed her family until the end of the week. In a bleak social environment, smoking may be her single pleasure. Some groups may be fearful about what the medical profession might do. For example, Afro-Caribbeans with mental health problems may have a fear of being too readily labelled as having serious mental illnesses.

## Techniques for assessing the needs of hard to read groups

- *Routine data sources.* Additional and unexpected data sources may be available from local authority housing or social services departments. Special analyses of the census data may be requested from the local public health department. This will provide some information about the ethnic origin of householders as well as the more familiar socioeconomic data.
- *Snowballing.* This is a technique whereby people with particular characteristics identify other people who may provide useful information. It is a technique which has been used for drug misusers and is described in detail by Griffiths et al.[15] Some workers have also found the technique useful in identifying the health issues as seen by ethnic minority elders.
- *Specific registers.* To some groups, lists smack of a totalitarian state and may reinforce some of the fears identified earlier. Local authorities may have lists of travellers. Some practices in parts of the country will already have their own registers. It may be worth setting up or extending an existing register as an investment for health needs work in the future. This will be of particular relevance to practices with significant numbers of patients with identifiable needs. It may be possible to search the practice list

for certain surnames. This has been done in studies of the needs of ethnic minorities.

● *Collecting information.* Some writers have argued that conventional techniques such as written questionnaires are appropriate in many circumstances. Response rates can be greatly improved by involving members of the community in the design and administration of such questionnaires. Focus groups and semistructured interviews are also well described techniques which have a place in looking at the needs of minority groups.

## Monitoring change and evaluation

It is essential, at the outset of any project to decide how the success of any project will be measured. Any organisations providing funds will almost certainly require this type of information. Targets for achievement need to be realistic, challenging, and achievable. Practices are likely to be able to detail needs assessment projects in their practice annual report.

---

### Summary points

- Clarify objectives of your needs assessment project.
- Involve all members of the practice team.
- Involve the trusts.
- Involve the public.
- Identify external help and funding if required.
- Consider what any hard-to-reach groups are in your practice.
- Decide how the project will be reported and evaluated.

---

## References

1 Secretary of State for Health. *The New NHS* (Cm 3807). London: Stationery Office, 1997.
2 Secretary of State for Scotland. *Designed to care.* Edinburgh: Scottish Office, 1997.
3 Shanks J, Kheraj S, Fish S. Better ways of assessing health needs in primary care. *BMJ* 1995;**308**:480–1.
4 Del Mar, CB, Glasziou PP. Antibiotics for the symptoms and complications of sore throat. In: Douglas R, Bridges-Webb C, Glasziou P, Lozano J, Steinhoff M, Wang E, eds. *Acute respiratory infections module of the Cochrane database of systematic reviews* (updated 3 June 1997). Available in the Cochrane Library (database on disc and CD-ROM). The Cochrane Collaboration; Issue 3. Oxford: Update Software; 1997 (updated quarterly).

5 Lalonde M. *A new perspective on the health of Canadians. A Working Document.* Ottawa: Information Canada, 1974.
6 Williams R. Diabetes mellitus. In: Stevens A, Raftery J, eds. *Health care needs assessment.* Vol. 1. Oxford: Radcliffe Medical Press, 1994.
7 Murray SA, Graham LJC. Practice based needs assessment: use of four methods in a small neighbourhood. *BMJ* 1995;**310**:1443–8
8 Peckham S, Spanton J. Community development approaches to health needs assessment. *Health Visitor* 1994;**67**:124–5.
9 Mays N, Pope C. Observational methods in healthcare settings. *BMJ* 1995;**311**:182–4.
10 Gillam SJ, Murray SA. *Needs assessment in general practice.* Occasional Paper 73. London: Royal College of General Practitioners, 1996.
11 Frankel SJ. Health needs, health care requirements, and the myth of infinite demand. *Lancet* 1992;**337**:1588–9.
12 Hobbs FDR, Parle JV, Kenkre JE. Accuracy of routinely collected clinical data on acute admissions to one hospital. *Br J Gen Pract* 1997;**47**:439–40.
13 Harley K, Jones C. Quality of Scottish Morbidity Record (SMR) data. *Health Bulletin* 1996;**54**:410–17.
14 Gabbay M, Gabbay J. Assessing the needs of hard to reach groups. In: Harris A, ed. *Needs to know.* London: Churchill Livingstone, 1997.
15 Griffiths P, Gossop M, Powis B, Strang J. Researching hidden populations of drug users by privileged access interviewers: methodological and practical issues. *Addiction* 1993;**88**:1617–26.
16 Cox J, ed. *Rural general practice in the United Kingdom.* Occasional Paper 71. London: Royal College of General Practitioners, 1996.
17 Watt I, Franks AJ, Sheldon TA. Health and health care of rural populations in the UK: is it better or worse? *J Epidemiol Community Health* 1994;**48**:16–21.

# 5 Health needs assessment in primary care – II Practical issues and possible approaches

SCOTT A MURRAY and JOHN WILKINSON

Health care resources are increasingly in demand: needs assessment aims to ensure that they are targeted to improve the population's health in the most efficient way. This chapter offers a five-stage practical guide to help primary care groups as set out in the NHS white papers,[1,2] and also individual general practitioners assess the needs of their respective populations before proceeding with providing or commissioning services to meet those needs. Historically much service provision has been service- rather than needs-led, provided as before and at the convenience of providers rather than patients. The needs of patients are described as being central to the way in which the new NHS will operate. General practitioners, primary care managers, and departments of public health are seeking the help of an explicit framework to hold together different aspects of need, and to help prioritise and action changes. This paper outlines an approach which is feasible for individual practices, groups of practices, and for populations around 100 000 people (typically the size of the new primary care groups described in the Government's White Paper).

The process of health needs assessment (HNA) can be carried out at different *levels* (from international down to individual patient), can use different *approaches* at each level (from global to

47

specific diseases), and can use a mix or "toolbox" of *methods* at each level.

## What approach to HNA is relevant to my situation?

### A global approach

It makes sense to take an initial overview of the health and social needs of the population group you serve, to identify which of a variety of interventions might be best to undertake on behalf of your patients to improve their health and well-being. This global approach might, for example, help general practitioners prioritise which of the many disease guideline documents they are currently receiving should be adopted next, according to patient needs and capacity to benefit. Issues relating to the wider determinants of health can be taken to the relevant agencies for action – in London and in Edinburgh bus routes have been changed and play areas developed!

### A focused approach

Such an approach may concentrate on:

- a speciality, for example, mental health;
- a disease, for example, epilepsy, Alzheimer's disease, cerebral palsy;
- a client group, for example, the elderly, single mothers, the unemployed, farmers;
- a group with a need for interventions, for example, people waiting for an orthopaedic appointment, or physiotherapy;
- vulnerable groups of patients, for example, ethnic minorities;
- patients who are socially deprived, to address issues of inequity.

## What methods of assessing needs are most suitable in my situation?

Different information sources and methods of investigating give complementary insights into health needs generally. Concentrate on gathering the information that will give you the most useful insights, rather than on collecting all sorts of information whether useful or not. A locally appropriate mix of methods can use data from various sources such as:

- practice-held information, accessing computer records, and "soft" information from all members of the PHCT(s); good for assessing ongoing physical problems;
- routinely available local statistics from hospitals, and the census;
- public consultation exercise using focus groups, rapid appraisal, or other methods of interacting with local people; good for uncovering problems relating to drug abuse, HIV, and social issues;
- a postal survey; good for providing data about acute illness in the community and suggestions for changes to services; a covering letter by the patient's general practitioner may improve the return rate.

For instance, the needs of people with mental health problems have been assessed at small area level using three of the above methods.[3] Detailed guidance on practical aspects is now available including a workbook and a "rough guide".[4-7]

## Getting started

### Who should assess needs?

Most approaches can be undertaken by an individual or a group. Although group work is more difficult to organise, there are major benefits. Group members who work in the community have valuable knowledge of local needs, and will feel an ownership of the results if they have been involved. Practice staff involved may require additional resources or locum cover. Public health and primary care can contribute complementary skills and insights at every level. Dependent on funding, some aspects of needs assessment can be carried out by an external agency if the relevant skills or time is unavailable (for example, to carry out focus groups or a postal survey).

### How do you define the problem or area to be assessed?

Most practices and even locality groups will have little time to devote to needs assessment, and therefore it is important to target any effort in the most productive way. A first needs assessment project must deliver rapid success to stimulate those involved in order to progress further. In a few practices, the issues that need to be tackled will be very obvious – perhaps in an area of inner city deprivation. However, for most practices, the priorities will vary depending on the demographic profile, common illnesses, and social needs. Consider the frequency, impact, and costs of different diseases. Priorities might be reached by asking the following questions:

- Is there a realistic chance of achieving change?
- Is the cost of undertaking the work proportional to the likely benefits?
- What are the priorities being suggested by other agencies, for example, health authority/board, social services?
- Does the practice or Primary Care Group wish to look at issues that are not directly under their control such as housing and transport?

## A five stage approach

### Stage 1 – Collect routine practice information

Routine data from general practices can highlight needs that are dealt with in primary care. The first box lists data, which give an overall practice perspective on needs. Ask your practice manager to collect as much as is reasonably available. Some computer software such as GPASS in Scotland has an interrogation facility whereby a practice profile can be generated automatically. This is especially useful in comparing practice data with other practices, or in collating data together in localities. Several networks exist in different parts of the country to optimise the use of such data.[8]

### Stage 2 – Collect hospital, community trust, and census data

Standard "routine" hospital use data do not routinely get fed back to practices. Thus the knowledge and understanding which most general practitioners have of the hospital services that their group of patients receive is limited. Although routinely collected clinical data may contain a number of inaccuracies,[9] the quality of some data bases has substantially improved.[10] Detailed hospital use

# Box 5.1   Stage 1 – Collect routine practice information

- Age sex profile in 5-year bands, males and females.
- Prescribing details:
  - repeat prescribing rates from practice computer;
  - collated prescribing figures (PACT or Scottish Prescribing Analysis).
- Prevalence of some specific chronic disease, for example, IHD, COAD, asthma, epilepsy, psychosis, thyroid disease, hypertension, and diabetes.
- Data from practices payment details:
  - percentage of patients attracting deprivation payments;
  - family planning uptake;
  - temporary residents;
  - obstetric care and other item of service payments.
- Health promotion and disease prevention data:
  - smoking, alcohol consumption, substance misuse, BMI data;
  - immunisation coverage levels (2- and 5-year-olds);
  - cervical cytology coverage.
- Contacts with general practitioners:
  - surgery consultation rate/1000 registered patients/year;
  - house call rate/1000;
  - out of hours visits/1000;
  - telephone advice/1000.
- Contacts with other members of PHCT:
  - practice nurse contacts/1000 patients/year;
  - health visitor contacts per/1000;
  - district nurse contacts per/1000.
- Knowledge (mostly implicit of the PHCT) of local health needs:
  - health visitor: practice profile, breast feeding rates, use of other agencies;
  - district nurse: workload details, observations in patients' homes;
  - practice nurse: workload details, for example influenza coverage rate;
  - receptionists: patients' perceptions, availability of appointments.
- Deaths – causes, place, preventable factors.
- Turnover of patients.
- Other sources – suggestions box, patient participation group.

*continued*

---

**Box 5.1 – *continued***

- Notes search may yield the following if thought useful:
  - incidence of acute illnesses and symptoms presenting;
  - telephone ownership percentage;
  - unemployment rate, domestic problems documented.

If reliable data (for example use of investigations, referrals ) are available from other sources, use these data rather than duplicate work in the practice for the following:

- Use of investigations (per 1000 patients per year, individually for bacteriology, virology, haematology, biochemistry, radiology, ECGs).
- Referrals to physiotherapy, chiropody, occupational therapy (per 1000 patients per year).
- Outpatient referrals per 1000.
- Attendance rate at accident and emergency department.
- Hospital admissions rate/1000.

---

can now be compared between practices and localities, facilitated by local public health departments. Such data must be interpreted carefully as demand and supply often have more influence on hospital use than need. Use of hospital services may not be a proxy for morbidity in the community.[11] The second box lists the variables that general practitioners working in Edinburgh South East Locality found most informative for understanding the current usage of hospital services by individual practices.

Health authorities and boards have also a range of census information available at small area level. This information is extremely useful to highlight social inequities at small area level, such as in an underprivileged housing estate. Jarman and Townsend scores may be available, but at practice or locality level the six census parameters in this box may be sufficient to give a view of social need. It is vital to request very specific, interesting summary data from the health authority or board, otherwise you will be swamped with too much detail which will obscure the larger picture, and also be too lengthy for general practitioners to absorb.

At practice level such data can be presented at a practice-planning meeting and inform the annual practice business plan. In Edinburgh South East Locality the above data were fed back at a meeting to which one general practitioner from each practice

# Box 5.2  Stage 2 – Collect hospital, community trust, and census data

In each case a direct comparison with the district/boards figures give added understanding. In other neighbourhoods with different local needs, different data may be more relevant but this list is a point of departure.

| Statistics | Most useful variables |
|---|---|
| **In-patient data** | Ten most frequent diagnoses made at hospital inpatient discharge (rates per 1000 registered patients), tabulated in descending order* |
| | Elective admission (rate per 1000 residents) |
| | Non-elective admission (rate per 1000 residents) |
| | Average mean waiting time (days) |
| | Ten most frequent day case diagnoses per 1000 patients, tabulated in descending order of frequency |
| | Top three day-case procedures per 1000 patients, in descending order of frequency |
| **Out-patient data** | Out-patient referral rate per 1000 residents |
| | Referral rates for five most frequent specialities, tabulated in descending frequency |
| | Mean waiting time in days |
| | Attendances at A&E per 1000 patients |
| **Obstetric data** | Births (rate per 1000 registered patients) |
| **Community data** | District Nursing visits per 1000 patients per year |
| | Health Visitors, visits and clinic attendances per 1000 patients per year |
| **Investigations** | Use of investigations (per 1000 patients per year), for bacteriology, virology, haematology, biochemistry, radiology, ECGs |
| **Referrals** | To physiotherapy (per 1000 patients per year, clinic and domiciliary) |
| | To chiropody (per 1000 patients per year, clinic and domiciliary) |
| | To occupational therapy (per 1000 patients per year) |
| **Census** | Percentage of residents with limiting long term illness |
| | Demographic profile, in 5 year bands |
| | Unemployment rates, male and female (%) |
| | Percentage house owners |
| | Percentage car owners |
| | Percentage of households with lone parents |

* The ICD 10 codes to three digits are recommended, transfers are excluded, and patients with multiple discharges from the same hospital, using the same facility and with the same diagnosis, are counted only once.

was invited. Protected time and hence a good attendance was gained by the availability of a fee from the general practice fundholding management allowance to all attendees. Under the new arrangements, after the abolition of fundholding, it should be possible to undertake similar exercises with the use of management allowances associated with the new Primary Care Groups. This data highlighted considerable variations in the use of inpatient, outpatient, and community services such as nursing and chiropody, with the two most common reasons for admission – termination of pregnancy and dental caries – both preventable. The general practitioners after presentation of the data and discussion left written comments on what they found most interesting about their practice, suggestions to improve or extend the data, and how the data could be used by individual practices and the locality. Subsequent meetings are planned to gain other perspectives of need in the locality from the other data sources mentioned above.

### Stage 3 – Gaining public involvement

Health professionals define "needs" in terms of services that they can provide, whereas patients may have a different perception of what would make them healthier: a job, a bus route to the shops, or some benefits advice, for example. Thus patient and public interaction and input is vital to gain an "honest consumer perspective". This can be obtained by the use of one or more of the following methods:

- interviews with patients;
- informal discussions with voluntary groups or a community health council, for example;
- suggestion boxes;
- complaints procedures;
- health forum;
- focus groups with the elderly or people with diabetes, for example;
- rapid appraisal.

Details about the last two of these methods are contained in the third box.

# Box 5.3   Stage 3 – Gaining public involvement

## Focus groups

Focus groups are facilitated discussion groups which allow the members of the target population to express their ideas in a spontaneous manner that is not structured by the researcher's predetermined ideas. They can give useful insights into perceived needs, quality of services, and understandings of health issues. They can raise issues which are important to patients, but do not give quantifiable information. Initial training is required to facilitate focus groups, and a variety of different groups may be necessary to be representative in some situations. For further details see "Introducing focus groups" in reference 11.

*Practical points*
- The optimum size for a group is between 8 and 12 participants.
- The facilitator introduces topics for discussion.
- Proceedings are recorded on tape and later transcribed, or in note form, preferably by another facilitator.

## Rapid appraisal

A team ideally with a mixture of professional insights gathers data about both needs and resources in the area under study from:

- interviews with key informants (individuals with knowledge of the community because of their job or social position) and patients;
- available documents about the neighbourhood/community;
- observations made inside homes and in the neighbourhood.

*Practical points*
Use the framework of an information pyramid to guide collection and analysis.[12]

- Collate the perceived needs, priorities and community perceived solutions for each box of the information pyramid.
- Consider facilitating change in primary care services, commissioning of secondary care, and local advocacy to improve wider determinants of health.

## Stage 4 – Undertake (or use an existing) postal survey

Surveys to assist local decision-making processes must be modestly defined and use a mixture of lay and medical concepts. Computerised search and mail merge facilities allow most practices to send questionnaires (with covering letters and reply-paid envelopes) to specific patient groups. A well-conducted postal survey of a representative sample can give a reliable estimate of the true burden of morbidity in the population, and may inform contract specification. Assistance will normally be needed to select an instrument or to design one, and with sampling and data analysis. A variety of validated instruments for generic and disease-specific surveys are available.[14] Questions concerning the areas

---

**Box 5.4   Stage 4 – Undertake (or use an existing) postal survey**

Surveys to assist local decision-making processes must be modestly defined and use a mixture of lay and medical concepts. Questions concerning the areas below may be especially relevant, and consider also checking a sample of medical records from non-respondents.

- Acute illnesses and experience of common symptoms
- Use of health services over the last 6 or 12 months
- Patient satisfaction
- Perceived need for current and potential services
- Specific concerns and worries which may affect health
- Consider a general health status instrument, for example SF36, SF12
- Consider a disease-specific instrument
- Specific questions for people with specific long term health problems or carers
- Chronic illness*
  - any long term illness
  - several marker conditions, for example hypertension, back pain
- Social and demographic characteristics*
  - car or house ownership, unemployment

* May not be necessary if data obtained already

---

outlined in the next box may be especially relevant, as such data may not be obtained easily from other sources.

## Stage 5 – Collation of the information from the different sources

*At practice level*

Present the major findings of each method to a meeting attended by as many of the practice team as possible, and discuss what changes should be made to the established work patterns and services that the practice offers. New initiatives identified should be prioritised and incorporated in the practice business plan for the coming year. Feedback can be given to the local hospitals and community trusts if relevant.

*At locality level (Primary Care Group)*

As the stages of the needs assessment may take a number of months, present the major findings of each method as they become available. Protected time is vital for practice representatives to study the information together, starting to get a feel for the needs of the locality as the complementary data builds up. A specific meeting, possibly facilitated by the local public health department, will be important to prioritise the suggestions raised by the various data. Techniques for prioritising needs include the nominal group technique, and use of a ranking matrix can give useful structure to such meetings. With the nominal group technique, needs or interventions are listed, discussed, then ranked by each participant until an agreed level of consensus is reached. This encourages debate and quick decisions can be made. To use a ranking matrix, criteria for priority interventions are defined, such as potential to improve health, capacity to implement, and equity implications. Participants score each potential intervention for each criterion, and the scores are totalled.[15]

Health needs assessment is a cyclical process. Needs change over time. You should try as best as you can to evaluate how well needs have been met. This will bring you back to assessing the needs that have not been met by your action (Figure 5.1).

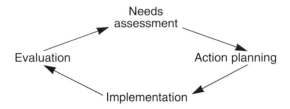

*Figure 5.1   Cyclical process of health needs assessment.*

## How realistic is assessment of health needs in primary care?

Lack of planning time and the pressure to respond to the immediate needs of patients has prevented up until now needs assessment in primary care. The fundholding initiative, emphasising efficient purchasing of services, has not championed needs assessment and has largely ignored non-health service aspects of health needs. The advent of locality commissioning and the creation of Primary Care Groups will now allow some general practitioners protected time and enable liaison with public health departments for assessing the needs of their practices. This strategic work is realistic and possible and has the potential to make primary care more effective at improving health by targeting available resources but resources and training will be necessary for this to work.

---

### Summary points

- A practical strategy for assessing local health needs is required.
- This approach uses practice-held data, routinely available local statistics, a patient/public consultation exercise, and (possibly) a postal survey to gain various perspectives on need.
- Request and obtain very specific, useful summary data, otherwise you will be swamped with details which obscure the larger picture.
- Collate the information, assess priorities, and plan and evaluate changes.
- Time and resources must be available at practice and primary care group level.

---

# References

1 Secretary of State for Health. *The New NHS* (Cm 3807). London: Stationery Office, 1997.
2 Home and Health Department. *Designed to care.* Edinburgh: Scottish Office, 1997.
3 Murray SA, Chick J, Perry B. Mental health, alcohol and drugs: constructing a community profile. *Primary Care Psychiatry,* 1996;2:237–43.
4 Harris A. *Needs to know: a guide to needs assessment for primary care.* London: Churchill Livingston, 1997.
5 Gillam S, Murray SA. *Needs assessment in general practice.* Occasional Paper 73. London; Royal College of General Practitioners, 1996.
6 Hooper J, Longworth P. *Health needs assessment in primary care. A workbook for primary health care teams.* Calderdale and Kirklees Health Authority, 1997.
7 Scottish Needs Assessment Programme. *A rough guide to needs assessment in primary care.* Glasgow: Scottish Needs Assessment Programme, 1998.
8 Smith N, Wilson A, Weekes T. Use of Read Codes in the development of a standard database. *BMJ* 1995;311:313–15.
9 Hobbs FDR, Parle JV, Kenkre JE, Accuracy of routinely collected clinical data on acute medical admissions to one hospital. *Br J Gen Pract* 1997;47:439–40.
10 Harley K, Jones C. Quality of Scottish Morbidity Record (SMR) data. *Health Bulletin* 1996;54:410–17.
11 Payne JN, Coy J, Patterson S, Milner PC. Is use of hospital services a proxy for morbidity? A small area comparison of the prevalence of arthritis, depression, dyspepsia, obesity, and respiratory disease with inpatient admission rates for these disorders in England. *J Epidemiol Community Health* 1994;48:74–8.
12 Kitzinger J. Introducing focus groups. *BMJ* 1995;311:299–302.
13 Murray SA, Tapson J, Turnbull L, McCallum J, Little A. Listening to local voices: adapting rapid appraisal to assess health and social needs in general practice. *BMJ* 1994;308:698–700.
14 Wilkin D, Hallam L, Dogget M. *Measures of need and outcomes in primary health care.* Oxford: Oxford Medical Publications, 1992.
15 Annett H, Rifkin SB. *Guidelines for rapid participatory appraisal to assess community health needs: a focus for health improvements for low-income urban and rural areas.* Geneva: WHO, 1995.

# 6 Whose priorities? Listening to patients and professionals

JOANNE JORDAN, THERESE DOWSWELL,
STEPHEN HARRISON, RICHARD J LILFORD,
and MAGGIE MORT

External inputs to health needs assessment and the prioritisation of health services may be seen as one means of addressing the "democratic deficit" of which the NHS has become increasingly guilty. Such external inputs can be discussed in respect of three levels. The first, which is not further discussed in this chapter, concerns the formal governance arrangements of the service, and encompasses questions about the possible election of health authority members and the possible transfer of the NHS purchasing function to local government authorities.[1,2] The second level of input may be characterised by arrangements for consultation with the general public, irrespective of whether they happen to be current patients or users. The third level concerns the consultation of current users about needs and priorities. In this chapter we concentrate on these latter two levels, the importance of which has recently been given recognition in the new white paper *The New NHS: modern, dependable.*[3]

What follows is divided into three sections. The first outlines the main methods which health authorities have recently employed to consult their local publics about matters such as service priorities, and discusses some of the most important implications that arise from the different constructions of "the public" entailed by these. The second section discusses the reactions of NHS managers and senior professionals to health care user groups. The final section considers broader issues raised for health needs assessment, with

60

particular emphasis on the challenges posed for a primary care-led NHS.

## Health authority consultation of the public

Whilst recent research on the nature and extent of public involvement activities has found the amount to have increased over earlier levels, the quality of consultation remains questionable.[4,5] Although some health authorities have established ongoing consultation procedures, including citizens' juries, large-scale postal panels and smaller face-to-face panels, the bulk has tended to be relatively inconsistent, exemplified by one-off surveys of the public or consultation with local user groups. Moreover, the majority of authorities continue to have no on-going means of consultation in place.[4]

These approaches may be classified according to two simple dimensions.[4] One dimension relates to whether or not respondents to the consultation exercise were provided with any *information*, whilst the second relates to whether respondents were able to engage in any discussion or *deliberation* in arriving at their views. These dimensions define the matrix shown as Table 6.1.

Table 6.1  Typology of approaches to public consultation on health care priorities

|  | Informed | Uninformed |
| --- | --- | --- |
| Deliberated | Citizen's juries User consultation panels (for example, Somerset panels) | Focus groups |
| Undeliberated | Questionnaire surveys with written information | Opinion surveys of standing panels/one-off questionnaires |

Citizens' juries[6] and similar panels of members of the public[7] place respondents in the situation where they are informed about the issues and choices at stake, and must deliberate with others in order to arrive at a recommendation. It might be said therefore that such mechanisms attempt to collect the views of the public not necessarily as they are, but as they might be if information and the opportunity for discussion were available. Diametrically opposed is an approach which seeks to consult the public as it is,

61

usually on the basis of statistically representative sampling. Such opinion surveys collect data from a generally uninformed public and do not encourage deliberation. The other two cells of Table 6.1 are hybrids; focus groups encourage discussion of uninformed opinion, while there are a very small number of cases where attempts have been made to provide survey respondents with a written briefing.

Either construction of the public, uninformed/undeliberating or informed/deliberating is open to objection, and of course any such objection can be used by NHS "insiders" as a pretext for ignoring or overriding the outcomes of consultation. It is clear that the organisers of consultation exercises can help to produce the outcomes that they prefer by the choice of question(s) posed, though this can be avoided through the involvement of the public in the formulation of the enquiry.

Whilst some studies have found former jury and panel participants to be satisfied with their experience and to express the view that ordinary people can, in general, participate effectively in such exercises,[8] the findings from other research suggest that opinion survey respondents are reluctant to accept a public role in health care prioritisation.[9] This suggests that informed/deliberating mechanisms may be as valuable as processes for enhancing participation as for producing substantive recommendations.

## Responding to user groups

In addition to the procedures for consultation outlined above, health authorities can opt to involve existing user groups. Where this has occurred research suggests that it is based on an essentially pragmatic acceptance of the groups as legitimate stakeholders in health care decision-making as health authorities are influenced by legislative change and occasionally by strong personal commitment to user led services.[10] Often, a strong feature of this recognition is officials' need for better information about both existing services and needs and priorities identified by the groups. In this context, user groups are seen as excellent conduits of information where there is a growing recognition that managers and professionals do not necessarily "know best".

However, having recognised the legitimate role of user groups, officials can be quick to qualify and circumscribe their influence, typically through a questioning of the groups' "representativeness".

This ambivalence is part of a more encompassing approach in which officials are able to undermine the legitimacy of groups should the perceived need arise,[1] while, at the same time, employ the user groups' views in their own negotiations with other officials.[11]

## Primary care consultation of the public

The preceding paragraphs have confirmed, albeit limited, attempts to involve the public in health care decision making. Given that official attention has been most keenly focused on the need and opportunity for health authority local consultation,[12] it is no surprise that the vast majority of initiatives have occurred at this level. Meanwhile relatively little attention has been paid to specifically primary care local consultation.[13] Whilst it may have been possible in the past to minimise the need for primary care involvement in such activity, recent and on-going policy developments make this argument now largely redundant. Above all, the increasing role of primary care, latterly in purchasing, and most likely in future locality-based commissioning of health services, makes the need to determine and respond to specifically *local* needs particularly acute.[12,14]

Although these developments set up the appropriateness of local health needs assessment as a basis of purchasing and commissioning they do not in themselves make *local participation* in such assessment requisite. Indeed, there are numerous ways of assessing the health needs of a local population, many of which do not entail going anywhere near the population itself.[15] The remainder of this section therefore discusses why primary care practitioners should involve the local community in decision making about health care provisioning and, importantly, considers the obstacles to such participation.

While the idea that GPs, in particular, are in a position to act as proxies for patient need is currently prominent,[16] two related issues make this assumption questionable. First, the evidence suggesting differing perceptions of doctors and patients[17,18] and secondly, the disparity between demand versus needs.[19,20] Taken together, these highlight the danger of assuming knowledge about the distribution of health (need) in a community based on practice experience alone. However, not only does it appear that many health professionals, including GPs, continue to view the proactive seeking out of need as necessarily secondary to a primary care responsibility for individual demand, but also they see local knowledge as frequently "inferior" to that generated by clinical observation and diagnosis.[21,22] As the majority of illness experience does not lead to a medical consultation,[23] professional knowledge cannot, however, be assumed to reflect individual experience, and presentation at surgery may best be understood as one expression of demand. One way of effectively filling gaps in understanding is therefore to consult the local community.

The issue of equity in health (provision) also makes it incumbent to move beyond a model of primary care based on professional response to demand to one which recognises the importance of responding to, otherwise unidentified, need. Contrary to the received wisdom concerning the positive relationship between level of economic development and health status, there is increasing evidence that it is the *distribution* and *degree* of inequality in economic welfare that has a direct impact on health.[24] Although local participation in health care decision making can run the danger of increasing this inequality (by allowing those most able to register their demands or needs to do so at the expense of the less articulate)[25] nevertheless, handled appropriately, previously marginalised groups can be provided with both a voice and a means of active involvement in health care decision-making.[26] The box below shows some typical methods of public consultation.

## Current potential for primary care consultation

Following this brief consideration of the imperative for local consultation, what scope exists for such activity under current health care policy and organisation? As already mentioned, problems arise from the fact that not only is primary health care essentially demand driven, but this demand is also arbitrarily divided into practice specific populations which may, but more often do not, correspond to naturally occurring geographical localities and populations.[13] In terms of the practical implications for community-based health needs assessment, a fundamental shift in both professional and official thinking is therefore required, towards an acknowledgement in both the organisation and funding of primary care the appropriateness of responding to local (as distinct from practice) population need.[27,28]

The poor understanding and limited uptake of local consultation within primary care[21,29] must, at least, in part arise from the absence

---

## Box 6.1 Methods of public consultation

| | |
|---|---|
| **Citizen's juries** | Participants selected as representatives of public/local opinion. Juries sit for a specified length of time during which time they are presented with information to help in decision-making. Typically, experts give evidence and jurors have an opportunity to ask questions/debate relevant issues.[6] |
| **User consultation panels** | Consist of number of local people, selected as representative of locality/population. Typically, involve member rotation to ensure a broad range of views is heard. Topics for consideration are decided in advance and members are presented with relevant information in order to encourage informed discussion. Meetings often facilitated by moderator.[7] |
| **Focus groups** | Typically, semistructured moderator-led discussion groups, with focus on specific topic(s). Usually involves between six and eight participants. Encourage debate and discussion. |
| **Questionnaire surveys** | Can either be postal or given out, for example, in surgery. Structured or systematic means of data collection which allows information to be collected from large sample of respondents Allows examination of relationship between variables. Most appropriately used when issues relevant to topic being investigated are already known in some detail. |
| **Opinion surveys of standing panels** | Standing panels are large scale (typically 1 000 upwards) sociologically representative samples of a health authority population who are surveyed at periodic intervals on matters of concern to the authority. There is usually a replacement policy aimed at ensuring that individuals do not serve on the panel for an indefinite period. |

---

of relevant training. What is an inherently challenging activity therefore becomes even more difficult. Working with a variety of groups representing different community interests demands considerable skills and flexibility for which health professionals are currently poorly prepared.[26] Not only must they acquire confidence in their own ability but local people may not be used to having their opinions invited, let alone being asked to undertake a more active role.[30] Consequently, not only are one-off consultation initiatives likely to have limited benefit in themselves, they may actively work against longer term effectiveness since the latter depends on proper structures and mechanisms for sustained, meaningful communication and action.

Despite the difficulties, there is already considerable scope for the development of community-based health needs assessment within primary care. Members of the wider primary health care team, in particular, are often already in touch with local networks, including resident's associations, mother and toddler groups, schools, and other voluntary organisations.[31] In addition, community nurses have long been responsible for the production of community profiles which could, for example, be used to develop stronger links with the community.[13] Not only does the spread of appropriate knowledge and skills as well as the practical need to divide any workload make it vital to involve the whole primary care team, but such involvement is in line with the underlying general ethos of full *participation* in health care decision making.[32]

One overriding issue remains. Comprehensive health needs assessment is likely to produce a wide range of different, potentially conflicting needs.[15,33] How are these different priorities, views and opinions to be weighed against one another in order to avoid a position of stalemate and to effect positive change? Available suggestions may differ but all are acutely aware of resource limitations and their implications for meeting the full range of need identified through any health needs assessment process.[33,34] There are no easy answers, but with regard to local involvement at least it is clear that people must be involved in the identification of need and, importantly, in the process by which these needs are prioritised and response effected.[26]

There is no doubt that the concept and practice of local participation in health needs assessment is particularly challenging. Although there are no ready-made models for how to go about it and there exists a number of potential obstacles, nevertheless there is already considerable potential for existing arrangements to be extended to incorporate local participation. Although it has been argued[24] that the recent policy obsession with needs assessment has been prompted by a desire to reduce public expenditure, this should not detract from the possibility of using needs assessment, particularly that premised on community involvement, as a means of not only promoting good health but also of reducing inequalities in its distribution.

---

## Summary points

- This article explores important issues associated with involving users and the public in health care decision making, with particular emphasis on the implications for health needs assessment.
- Although health authorities have increased local consultation in recent years, its quality remains dubious, with greatest emphasis on on-off consultation exercises.
- An ambivalence surrounding the information gained via public consultation means that views expressed may either be marginalised or incorporated according to professional priorities.
- The need to acknowledge limitations to professional knowledge as well as to respond to inequalities in health is emphasised and suggestions made as to how such a response can be effected utilising local knowledge.
- While a number of barriers to effective community based health needs assessment are identified, significant scope for greater local involvement in decision making currently exists.
- However, it is concluded that, in the longer term, appropriate changes to the organisation and funding of primary care are vital if effective involvement is to be sustained over time.

---

## References

1 Harrison S. The political and administrative centre should have an increased role in making health care rationing decisions: against the proposition. *BMJ* 1997;**314**:970–3.
2 Hunter DJ, Harrison S. Democracy, accountability and consumerism. In: Iliffe S, Munro J, eds. *Healthy choices: future options for the NHS*. London: Lawrence and Wishart, 1997.
3 Department of Health. *The New NHS: modern, dependable*. London: Secretary of State for Health, 1997.
4 Mort M, Harrison S, Dowswell T. Public Health Panels in the UK: influence at the margins? Khan UA. ed. *Innovations in participation*. London: Taylor and Francis, forthcoming.
5 Pickard S, Williams G, Flynn R. Local voices in an internal market: the case of community health services. *Social Policy and Administration* 1995;**29(2)**: 135–49.
6 Lenaghan J, New B, Mitchell E. Setting priorities: is there a role for citizens' juries? *BMJ* 1996;**312**:1591–3.

7 Bowie C, Richardson A, Sykes W. Consulting the public about health care priorities. *BMJ* 1995;**311**:1155 8.
8 Dowswell T, Harrison S, Lilford RJ, McHarg K. Letter. *BMJ* 1995;**311**:1168–9.
9 Heginbotham C. Rationing. *BMJ* 1992;**304**:1168–9.
10 Barnes M, Harrison S, Mort M, Shardlow P, Wistow G. Users, officials and citizens in health and social care. *Local Government Policymaking* 1996;**22**:9–17.
11 Mort M, Harrison S, Wistow G. The user card: picking through the organisational undergrowth in health and social care. *Contemporary Politics* 1996; **2**:1133–40.
12 NHS Management Executive. *Local voices, the views of local people in purchasing for health.* London: Department of Health, 1992.
13 Peckham. S. Local voices and primary health care. *Critical Public Health* 1992; **5**(2):36–40.
14 NHS Executive. *Developing NHS Purchasing and GP Fundholding.* EL (94) 79. London: Department of Health, 1994.
15 Gillam SJ, Murray SA. *Needs assessment in general practice.* Occasional Paper 73. London: Royal College of General Practitioners, 1996.
16 Department of Health and the Welsh Office. *General practice in the National Health Service: a new contract.* London: HMSO, 1989.
17 Heritage Z. *Community participation in primary care.* Occasional Paper 64. London: Royal College of General Practitioners, 1994.
18 Barnes M, Wistow G. Understanding user involvement. In: Barnes M, Wistow G, eds. *Researching user involvement.* Leeds: Nuffield Institute for Health Services Studies, 1992.
19 Bradshaw JR. A taxonomy of social need. In Mclachlan G, ed. *Problems and progress in medical care.* Oxford: Nuffield Provincial Hospital Trust, 1972.
20 Stevens A, Gabbay J. Needs assessment, needs assessment. *Health Trends* 1991; **23**(1):20–3.
21 Jordan J, Wright J, Wilkinson J, Williams R. *Health needs assessment in primary care: a study of understanding and experience in three districts.* Leeds: Nuffield Institute for Health, 1995.
22 Bowling A, Jacobsen B, Southgate L. Health Services priorities. Exploration in consultation of the public and health professionals on priority setting in an inner London health district. *Social Sci Med* 1993;**37**:851–7.
23 Last JM. The iceberg: completing the clinical picture in general practice. *Lancet* 1963;**2**:28–31.
24 Bradshaw J. The conceptualisation and measurement of need. In: Popay J, Williams G, eds. *Researching the people's health.* London: Routledge, 1994.
25 Percy-Smith J, Sanderson I. *Understanding local needs.* London: Institute for Public Policy Research (IPPR): Premier Printers, 1992.
26 Dockery G. Rhetoric or reality? Participatory research in the National Health Service. In: Koning CD and Martin, M, eds. *Participatory research in health.* London: Zed Books Ltd, 1996.
27 Jordan J, Wright J. Making sense of health needs assessment. *Br J Gen Pract*, 1997.**48**;695–6.
28 Ruta DA, Duffy MC, Farquharson A, *et al.* Determining the priorities for change in primary care: the value of practice-based needs assessment. *Br J Gen Practice* 1997;**47**:353–7.
29 Pritchard P. Community involvement in a changing world. In: Heritage Z, ed. *Community participation in primary care.* London: Royal College of General Practitioners, 1994.
30 Dowswell T, Drinkwater C, Morley V. Developing an inner city health resource centre. In: Heritage Z, ed. *Community Participation in primary care.* London: Royal College of General Practitioners, 1994.

31 Findlay G, Palmer J. Reorientating health promotion in primary care to participative approaches. In: Heritage Z, ed. *Community participation in primary care*. London: Royal College of General Practitioners, 1994.
32 Brown I. The organisation of participation in general practice. In: Heritage Z, ed. *Community participation in primary care*. London: Royal College of General Practitioners, 1994.
33 Robinson J, Elkan R. *Health needs assessment, theory and practice*. London: Churchill Livingstone, 1996.
34 London Health Economics Consortium and SDC Consulting. *Local health and the vocal community: a review of developing practice in community based health needs assessment*. London: London Primary Health Care Forum, 1996.

# 7 Health needs assessment in developing countries

JOHN WRIGHT and JOHN WALLEY

Historically the development of health services in most developing countries has been dominated by Western models of health care. These have rarely taken into account how local people explain illness, seek advice or rely on traditional healing methods. The emphasis has been on hospitals and curative care rather than trying to address local health needs equitably and effectively. Since the Alma Ata declaration on primary health care more attention has been given to increasing coverage of basic services and prevention of common diseases. However, the bias in resource allocation towards secondary care and urban areas remains.

Health needs are changing and new challenges from chronic diseases and HIV infection must be faced. Better coverage of preventive and essential health care services has led to greater emphasis on improving the quality of health care and ensuring that the most efficient use is made of scarce resources. For example, infant mortality has fallen dramatically in the last two decades, through child survival interventions such as oral rehydration for diarrhoea and immunisation programmes. With fewer children dying there has been greater emphasis on the need to tackle the causes of infant and child morbidity. Families can be smaller and this has highlighted the need improve the availability of family planning.

If health services are to address the changing health needs of their local populations, then planners and managers need useful and timely information about the health status of these populations. Some of this information can come from routine data sources or may be collected from large, one-off population studies. Some information can be obtained from community surveys.

## Routine information

Information about diseases or use of health services can help to build up a picture of the health needs of a local population.[1] Such epidemiological information can come from national, regional, or local sources:

- National census data can provide information on the age and sex distribution of a population. This information can be used to calculate crude birth rates and fertility rates.
- Death certification and registers can provide information on the cause and place of death. Infant mortality rates can be calculated from the number of liveborn infants who die in the first 12 months of life.
- Hospital in-patient records can be used to obtain numbers of admissions, cause of admission, length of stay (Figure 7.1).
- Out-patient consultations for numbers of patients and diagnoses.
- Disease notification systems can provide information on important infectious diseases.
- Maternity unit statistics can describe births rates, maternal ages and parity, numbers of low birth weight (less than 2500 g) babies and maternal mortality rates.
- Pharmacy information on the use of essential and non-essential drugs.
- Laboratories can provide information on the appropriate use of tests and numbers of positive tests (for example, sputum samples for pulmonary TB, malaria blood slides).
- Workplaces can provide data on absences due to sickness, occupational injuries, and regular employment health checks.

When considered in isolation this information provides a snapshot of a population's health. However, without comparative information this will be of limited use in planning health services. Comparison can be with other populations (national or regional) or with the same population over time.

The disadvantage of routine information is that it is often inaccurate, incomplete, and out of date. For example, out-patient records may only give the main complaint of patients attending, and may not distinguish new patient visits from repeat visits.

71

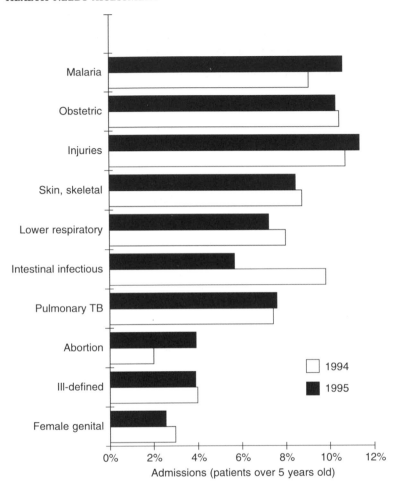

*Figure 7.1  Top ten causes of admission over two years, all hospitals Mashonaland Central Province, Zimbabwe, 1994 and 1995 (excluding normal deliveries, which form 27 and 25% respectively).*

Notifiable diseases may be missed and when they are picked up they are often not reported. It is also difficult to make generalisations about a local population from routine data. For example, people who attend a hospital are more likely to reflect a more affluent and urban population. One-off studies can provide more detailed, relevant and accurate information on a specific topic (see the box below) but are time-consuming and costly.

---

## Box 7.1   Example of combining different methods of needs assessment[13]

Bacterial and tuberculous meningitis are an important cause of morbidity and mortality in developing countries despite the availability of effective treatment.

- *Epidemiological assessment.* A national study was undertaken in Swasiland to describe the epidemiology, clinical features, and outcomes of each case of meningitis admitted to hospital. The overall case fatality was found to be 42% in all ages and 63% in adults. Significant association was found with a period of drought and the increasing contribution of HIV infection was highlighted. The results also identified the age distribution and aetiology of meningitis in the country and allowed an assessment of the potential impact of immunisation programmes.
- *Community appraisal.* Semistructured interviews were carried out on a random sample of mothers attending a health centre. A focus group discussion was conducted with a purposefully selected group of health workers. These interviews identified educational needs about the awareness of symptoms, and the importance of prompt referral and treatment.
- *Action.* In an effort to reduce the high mortality from meningitis by reducing delays in treatment, a co-ordinated education campaign for the public and health workers was undertaken using posters and outreach teaching sessions.

---

## Community appraisals

These describe approaches to needs assessments that emphasise involvement of local people (see the box below). There are a confusing number of terms to describe similar methods: rapid evaluation methods, rapid appraisal methods, rapid community surveys, rapid rural appraisal, relaxed rural appraisal, participatory rural appraisal.[2-6] The development of rapid appraisal methods during the 1980s came in recognition of the time-consuming and rigid nature of traditional epidemiological and questionnaire surveys. Experience with these appraisal methods showed that when done well they provided valuable, reliable, and timely information on health status, knowledge, attitudes, and behaviours. More recently, emphasis has been placed on encouraging people to participate actively in their own appraisal (for example, participatory rural appraisal).[2-4] Many of the principles behind these techniques stem from the formative work of Paulo Freire in enabling oppressed people to understand and address their own educational needs.[7]

---

### Box 7.2   Steps in community appraisal

- Define aims of appraisal
- Identify community for assessment
- Identify study team and train in qualitative techniques
- Examine available information
- Define key questions and issues
- Pilot questions in interviews or questionnaires
- Identify key informants
- Choose and use appropriate methods
- Analyse information after each interview
- Write report and develop action plan

---

In community appraisals the assessors support and facilitate community understanding and action rather than just record information (see next box). Local communities can be empowered by the opportunity to participate in health planning and health workers have the opportunity to appreciate the perceived strengths and weaknesses of services.

The information collected in community appraisals is used to develop acceptable and sustainable programmes in partnership with the community. These may be programmes of health care, nutrition, or family planning that improve services for the community. The same methods can be used to monitor and evaluate the developments.

The methods used for appraisals vary, but emphasis is on qualitative techniques of interviewing and listening to people (see boxes below).[9]

The assessors need to have good listening skills, a recognition that communities know their own needs, and common sense in analysing the results. Some training is necessary to provide the assessors with the skills needed to undertake appraisal techniques and generate good quality and reliable findings. They must also beware of generating false hopes in the community for what can be achieved.

# Box 7.3 Community appraisal of the factors affecting participation in nutrition, health, and development in commercial farms in Zimbabwe[8]

The workers and their families on commercial farms are one of the most disadvantaged in Zimbabwe. A Farm Health Programme has been operating for 15 years in Mashonaland Central Province, including child health, preschool, and nutrition activities. Malnutrition in under 5-year-old children remains more common on the communal farms than elsewhere. Hence there is a need for a better understanding of the factors influencing nutrition, health, and development.

## Appraisal

Eight farms, ranging from well- to under-developed, were selected. Permission of each commercial farmer was requested by telephone and followed up by an explanatory letter delivered by hand. On each farm the commercial farmer or representative was interviewed.

Participants for group discussions were recruited randomly, requesting:

- 6–8 female workers with preschool children;
- 6–8 permanent male workers with preschool children; and
- 6–8 seasonal workers with preschool children.

Anyone who appeared to hold some kind of authority was tactfully removed from the group discussion, by asking them to assist in drawing the social map, which was drawn on the ground and then copied. The research investigated:

- knowledge, attitudes and practices relating to health;
- felt needs, priority problems, opportunities, and solutions;
- factors affecting communication;
- factors affecting participation in health activities;
- factors likely to assist or hinder an intervention programme.

## Results

Child nutrition was not viewed as a priority problem by farm workers or farm owners. Farm workers cited poor working conditions, working hours, low salaries, and lack of family food. Child health care came much lower on the priority rankings.

*continued*

---

**Box 7.3 – *continued***

The workers are fragmented community with no sense of belonging to a group. There is tension between permanent workers, with better conditions, and seasonal workers.

A unhealthy child is described as being dirty, sick, thin, eats cold food, has a pot belly, and is miserable. Contributory factors include parental fighting, inadequate food, sickness, lack of child care at home or at preschool.

Issues likely to influence participation *negatively* included *zvondo* – jealousy and mistrust amongst women. For example, not organising a cooking roster for the preschool, as they don't want the woman whose turn it is to cook to benefit from the food. Another example is past poor response by the commercial farmer to their efforts – having dug toilet pits the farmer failed to provide cement and a builder to finish the job.

---

The choice of subjects for questionnaires or interviews will determine how generalisable the results are. This sampling can be done randomly, systematically (for example, every fifth house in a village) or purposefully selecting *key informants* (people with expert knowledge, for example, patients, mothers, sex workers, chiefs, elders, church leaders, shop keepers, health workers, government officials). Care should be taken when selecting key informants that they reflect the range of different interest groups.

Ideally a combination of methods should be used when assessing health needs, for example, analysis of routine health data plus a questionnaire or focus group. This allows cross-checking and validation of results and it increases their relevance or generalisability to the study population. Routine population data can be superficial and inaccurate; however, it does allow a quantitative comparison with other population data. A small number of interviews may not provide opinions that represent those of the whole community; however, they do allow an understanding of what people's true priorities are.

Language and literacy barriers may occur when discussing complex health issues. A variety of techniques can be used to overcome these barriers in non-literate populations. They include community mapping, seasonal calendars, Venn (chappati) diagrams, and dramatisation techniques.[3,4] These visually based

---

**Box 7.4   Methods of community appraisal**

- Summarising existing information from routine sources or previous surveys. Example: causes of morbidity and mortality.
- Exit interviews after a clinic visit to obtain the patient's perspective on the quality of care and understanding of the health messages received. Example: children with diarrhoea, checking that their mothers understand how to make up ORS.
- Interviews with health worker. Example: to assess their perception of local needs. Interviews can be structured with a standard list of questions, or semistructured, with just a list of topics that need to be covered.
- Ranking of priorities or preferences. Example: asking local people to produce a "league table" of needs.
- Case note review and audit. Example: examining the recording of tasks and health education given to patients.
- Household survey to assess family health needs. Example: seasonal variation in food intake and accessibility to clean water.
- Focus group discussion to obtain the opinions of a specific population group. Example: a facilitator guides the group of purposefully selected informants through a framework of questions that aim to stimulate discussion and communication of opinions. An assistant takes notes of the discussion for later analysis.
- Direct observation of chosen indicators or behaviours. Example: the performance of health workers in communication or clinical skills.

---

methods provide opportunities for local people to explore and analyse their needs in their own terms and enhances their involvement in the assessment.[10]

## Emergency needs assessment

Quick decisions and actions are imperative in the aftermath of a disaster. The immediate, life-supporting needs after any major disaster are similar whether the cause is a gradual onset, such as drought, famine, or war, or a sudden onset, such as floods or earthquakes. These needs include: clean and adequate water and sanitation; adequate food rations; shelter, including clothing and blankets; essential medical care.[11] Information must be obtained not

---

**Box 7.5.  The constraints to directly observed treatment for TB in Pakistan**

- *Context.* The study was part of the preparation for the introduction of daily observed treatment (DOT). DOT is being promoted by WHO to improve compliance, cure rates, and reduce multidrug resistance, but increases the demands on patients and providers.
- *Aim.* To understand the access constraints faced by patients to health facilities.
- *Sample.* Patients attending the diagnostic centres, selected to ensure a range of age, sex, urban/rural and new/ retreatment cases.
- *Method.* An in-depth interview using a checklist was conducted at the health facility.
- *Results.* Very little information was given about the disease and the need for compliance with the six months of treatment or the risks of default. There was considerable fear of stigma, especially for unmarried women. Family support was limited from husbands and in-laws of women, but their own families would be supportive.
- *Action.* The content for health education of patients and family supporter was informed by the study. The limits to which patients could reasonably be expected to attend daily at health centres was defined in terms of time, distance, and travel costs.

---

only from government or other agencies (including, increasingly, the international media), but from the affected community. This community will have the capacity to help itself and any disaster response should build on these capacities.

Involving the community is essential in assessing the effects of the disaster and targeting vulnerable groups (young children, the elderly, pregnant women). It is also vital to avoid cultural problems. Some can be avoided with intelligence (such as sending pork products to Islamic countries). Others require more insight; for example, a famine relief programme ran into problems because the affected population, used to a staple of white maize, had strong traditional beliefs that the yellow maize being distributed was inedible and poisonous.[12]

The United Nations High Commission for Refugees has developed a simple needs assessment tool called people-orientated planning to help guide decisions about refugee needs (Which foods should be supplied? How should they be distributed? Who should live where? What are the critical medical needs? What are the cultural patterns of health care? How are target groups best reached?) This is approached through an analysis of the refugee population profile, activities, and use of resources.

In addition to considering immediate needs, it is important to plan for the future. A community dependent entirely on donor food supplies will be vulnerable when these are withdrawn, especially if normal food production is still disrupted. Good surveillance systems are also vital to monitor health and malnutrition. For example, anthropometric surveys of children in refugee camps or outreach clinics, measuring weight-for-height or mid-upper arm circumference, can provide valuable nutritional assessments.[11] Monitoring of infectious diseases such as measles can prompt timely immunisations.

## Global needs

So far we have discussed local health needs assessent. National and international health needs are also important in planning health services. Most assessments of the relative importance of different diseases are based on how many deaths they cause. This convention has certain merits: death is an unambiguous event, and the statistical systems of many countries routinely produce the data required. There are, however, many diseases or conditions that are not fatal but that are responsible for great loss of healthy life: examples are chronic depression and paralysis caused by polio. These conditions are common, can last a long time, and frequently lead to significant demands on health systems.

Global needs are represented by the global burden of disease. This burden of disease includes both morbidity and mortality. Morbidity can be considered according to the amount of disability, for example from blindness, and the mortality can be expressed in terms of life years lost. The needs can then be expressed through a combined measure of such as the "*disability-adjusted life year*" or DALY.[14]

The proportion of disability and loss of life varies from disease to disease so there will be more disability due to leprosy but more years of life lost from tuberculosis. Overall the global burden of disease, when calculated as DALYs, is made up from approximately two-thirds from years of life lost (mortality) and one-third from disability (morbidity).

DALYs can be used to rank diseases in order of magnitude of burden of disease in developing countries. The existing rankings can be compared with a prediction of the future[15] (Table 7.1). This demonstrates the scale of the demographic and epidemiological transition anticipated by the year 2020, with depression and traffic accidents as the biggest predicted burdens of disease.

Table 7.1   League of ill health: how the burden will change in the developing world

| Cause | Rank 2020 | 1990 |
|---|---|---|
| Depression | 1 | 4 |
| Road traffic accidents | 2 | 11 |
| Ischaemic heart disease | 3 | 8 |
| Chronic obstructive pulmonary disease | 4 | 12 |
| Cerebrovascular disease | 5 | 10 |
| Tuberculosis | 6 | 5 |
| Lower respiratory infections | 7 | 1 |
| War | 8 | 16 |
| Diarrhoeal diseases | 9 | 2 |
| HIV | 10 | — |

In 1990 measles and malaria were ranked 6th and 7th

DALYs should be interpreted with caution because of the assumptions that are made.[16] For example, the combination of discounting and age weighting means that an infant's death has the same number of DALYs as the death of a young adult. They are based on incomplete, internationally available data that may contain inaccuracies. The calculation of DALYs is based on specific diseases or disease groups. Many diseases have multiple outcomes, and interventions may reduce the burden for more than one disease. For example, treatment of diabetes will reduce the risk of stroke, coronary heart disease, and renal failure.

To date DALYs have been calculated globally and by WHO region. Attempts are being made to estimate the national disease burdan, as in Ghana; however, limitations in data make this a difficult task.

Despite these limitations, DALYs are the only data available that combine morbidity and mortality into a simple indicator of burden of disease. This can be used to identify current and future international health needs and plan essential national health services.[17]

## Acting on the assessment

The hardest part of any needs assessment is translating the results into policies and practices which will provide beneficial change. The involvement of health workers in techniques such as rapid or rural appraisal will encourage changes at an individual level. Local workshops can provide an opportunity to pass on the lessons learnt to other health workers. If this change is going to be sustainable and adaptable, then the appraisal should be a continuous process with on-going feedback. Implementation of strategic changes can be facilitated if the policymakers themselves are actively involved in the process.

## Acknowledgements

We are grateful to Anthony Zwi and Aad van Geldermalsen for their comments and advice, and to Margaret Haigh for her secretarial support.

## Appendices

### Medical information needs

As in developed countries, evidence of effectiveness is an essential component of needs assessment. Attempts are currently being made to improve access to research information and effectiveness information using the internet, including:

- UK Cochrane Centre: http://www.cochrane.co.uk
- South African Cochrane Centre: http://www.mrc.ac.za/mrcnews/march96/cochrane.htm
- International Network for the Availability of Scientific Publications: http://oneworld.org/inasp/network.html
- Global Health Network: http://www.pitt.edu/HOME/GHNet/GHNet.html

## Epi info

Epi info is a software package developed by the Centers for Disease Control in the United States. It allows easy questionnaire design (EPED), data processing, and analysis. The analysis module provides a user-friendly statistical package. It is considered public domain and may be freely copied. Its simplicity and free availability make it ideal for researchers in developing countries. (Contact: The Division of Surveillance and Epidemiologic Studies, Epidemiology Program Office, Centers for Disease Control, Atlanta, Georgia 30333, USA.)

---

## Summary points

- Timely and accurate information is essential if health services in developing countries are to meet the changing health needs of their populations.
- Routine health information can provide an epidemiologically based assessment of ill health and identify what health service are needed.
- Community appraisals can provide valuable patient insight into patients' needs as well as empowering communities by participation in the planning of local health services.
- Emergency health needs are similar whatever the disaster. Community involvement, good surveillance and foresight are an important part of meeting these needs.
- The global burden of disease can be represented by disability adjusted life years (DALYs). These can help to identify current and future internation health needs, and plan essential health services.

---

## References

1 Vaughan JP, Morrow RH. *Manual of epidemiology for district health management.* Geneva: World Health Organisation, 1989.
2 Cornwall A, Jewkes R. What is participatory research? *Soc Sci Med* 1995;**41**: 1667–76.
3 Chambers R. *Rural appraisal: rapid, relaxed and participatory.* Discussion paper 311. Brighton: Institute of Development Studies, 1992.
4 Chambers R. Participatory rural appraisal (PRA): analysis of experience. *World Development* 1994;**22**:1253–68.
5 Rahman MA, Fals-Borda O. A self-review of PAR. In: *Action and knowledge: breaking the monopoly with participatory action research.* London: Intermediate Technology Publications, 1991.

6 Reynolds J. *Primary health care management advancement programme: assessing community health needs and coverage*. Geneva: Aga Khan Foundation, 1993.
7 Freire P. *Pedagogy of the oppressed*. New York: The Seabury Press, 1968.
8 Adams L, Goche T, Marime W, Mungate B, Shamuyarira L. *Report of participatory rural appraisal*. Mashonaland Central Province, 1996.
9 World Health Organisation. *Rapid evaluation method guidelines for maternal and child health, family planning and other health services*. Geneva: WHO, 1993.
10 de Koning K, Martin M. *Participatory research in health. Issues and experiences*. Johannesburg: Zed Books, 1996.
11 Seaman J, ed. Disasters. *Tropical Doctor* 1991;**21**(suppl 1).
12 Wright J, Ford H. Another African disaster. *BMJ* 1992;**305**:1479–80.
13 Ford H, Wright J. The impact of bacterial meningitis in Swaziland: an 18 month prospective study. *J Epid Comm Health* 1994:**48**:276–80.
14 World Bank. *World development report 1993: investing in health*. New York: Oxford University Press, 1993.
15 Murray C. *Investing in health research & development*. Geneva: WHO, 1996.
16 Barker C, Green A. Opening the debate on DALYs. *Health Policy and Planning* 1996;**11**:179–83.
17 Bobadilla J-L, Cowley P, Musgrove P, Saxenian H. Design, content and financing of an essential national package of health services. *Bull World Health Org* 1994; **72**:653–6.

# 8 Clinical and cost effectiveness issues in health needs assessment

ANTHONY SCOTT and CAM DONALDSON

Health needs assessment needs economics. Resource scarcity ensures that not all needs can be met and so choices have to be made about which health needs to meet and to what extent. The economic framework applied to needs assessment attempts to quantify what is currently happening to the population of interest in terms of their use of resources (the "programme budget") and examines the changes in costs and benefits of options for change ("marginal analysis"). The latter can be in the form of comprehensive economic evaluation based on randomised trials or pragmatic approaches that can be used more readily by purchasers and general practitioners in conjunction with evidence from the literature. Although the comprehensive form of economic evaluation is preferred to the pragmatic, it is obviously not possible, and often not relevant, to conduct a randomised trial every time a purchaser needs to make a decision. Thus the pragmatic form is to be preferred to no economic evaluation at all.

Meeting health needs requires the use of scarce resources. This inescapable fact forms the basis for the economic approach to needs assessment. Although much has been written about the role of economics in needs assessment and although economic approaches (or at least the language of economics) are now being used more often, it is important to highlight the basis and potential usefulness of the economic approach, both of which are still often ignored.[1-3]

The aim of this chapter is to argue that "needs assessment needs economics" if benefits to patients and to populations are to be maximised from the resources available. Any decision to commit NHS resources to meet health needs should be subject to some form of economic analysis. The next section sets out in more detail the basis of the economic approach to needs assessment and illustrates how it can contribute with practical examples. The strengths and weaknesses of the economic approach will then be discussed.

## Why does needs assessment need economics?

Once a needs assessment has been conducted and "needs" have been measured, a choice must be made about which needs should be met. A choice is necessary because of scarce NHS resources (and scarce local authority resources which can also be used to meet health needs). There is simply not enough resources to meet all needs and never will be. The decision to invest resources in one area of need means that the opportunity to use those resources in meeting another need is given up. This is known as the concept of "opportunity cost" where "cost" is defined as the value of benefits forgone from using resources in one way rather than the next best alternative.

To maximise the amount of need that can be met by the limited resources it is therefore necessary to know the amount of need that is met by a specific health care intervention (that is, its effectiveness or "marginal met need") and the amount of resources used in meeting this need (that is, the cost). Thus evidence on costs and benefits of health care interventions should form a key aspect of any needs assessment. Following this, an important part of the economic approach is marginal analysis or the analysis of change. So if a new health care intervention is introduced, or an existing one is expanded or contracted, what are the *changes* in costs (that is, resources used) and benefits (that is, the amount of need met by the intervention)? If the marginal benefits are judged to be greater than what could be achieved by using the resources differently, then the intervention should go ahead. Such an approach makes explicit the need to compare alternatives, implying that assessments of total need or burdens of diseases, for example, are not useful in making decisions about whether to introduce, expand, or contract health care interventions.

In the past, economists have been fairly critical of burden of illness approaches to needs assessment.[4,5] For example, simple needs assessments have measured relative "need" according to relative mortality and morbidity of different diseases. This ranking of the burden of illness has in turn implied that priority (and therefore resources) should be devoted to those diseases with the highest rates of mortality and morbidity. This approach is encapsulated in documents such as the *Health of the Nation*. However, because such an approach ignores both the relative effectiveness of interventions in each disease area (that is, marginal met need) and ignores the relative (opportunity) costs of meeting need, it will not lead to the maximisation of benefits to patients (that is, the greatest reduction in health need) from the resources available. For example, chiropody for elderly people has been shown to represent "good" value for money, yet foot problems do not cause major mortality of morbidity and so would not rank highly under a burden of disease approach.[6] Thus the priorities implied by a ranking of conditions according to burden of illness is likely to be different from conditions ranked according to the effectiveness and cost of their associated health care interventions.

The advent of evidence based health care has meant that the concepts of clinical effectiveness and health gain (that is, marginal met need) are now integral parts of many health needs assessments, especially in a purchasing context. However, the measurement of resource use within such exercises, although more common than five years ago, is still rare.

## Applying the economic approach to health needs assessment

The economic approach, using the concepts of scarcity, opportunity cost and marginal analysis, has been implemented through economic evaluation and its more pragmatic derivative, programme budgeting and marginal analysis (PBMA). The purpose of this section is to outline these approaches (which should be regarded as complementary to other approaches to needs assessment).

The main point to emphasise about economic evaluation with respect to needs assessment is not the technical terminology or the specific types and how they differ (for example, cost-utility, cost-effectiveness, cost-minimisation analysis), but that the overall economic framework is used and applied to different choice situations. The key stages of the application of the economic framework are shown in the box below.

---

**Box 8.1   Key stages in applying the economic framework to needs assessment**

(1) Find out what is currently happening to patients (programme budgeting).

(2) Evaluate options for change (marginal analysis):
    (a) Specify alternatives by:
        (i) identifying candidates for more resources,
        (ii) identifying services which could be provided to the same level of effectiveness but at less cost, so releasing resources for (i);
        (iii) identifying services which, although effective, may be less effective per pound spent than candidates in (i).
    (b) Assess the changes in costs and changes in benefits of options identified in (i) to (iii)

(3) Increase investment in candidates in (i) and reduce investment for those identified in (ii) and (iii), if benefits (effectiveness) overall are likely to increase.

---

The aim of needs assessment is, presumably, to match resources to needs to ensure that as much need as possible is met. Epidemiology tends to approach this problem from the point of view of "needs" in terms of burdens and causes of disease. To see how the economic approach can fit in to needs assessment, it is useful to divide the process of needs assessment into two main stages: (1) finding out what is currently happening to a population or group of patients and (2) evaluating options for change so that benefits to patients, such as health gain, are maximised given the resources available.

## Programme budgeting: how do we know where we are going if we do not know where we are?

The first stage is where the traditional epidemiological approach to needs assessment has been applied. The contribution of economics to this stage is that of "programme budgeting".[7] This refers to the process of finding out how many health care resources are currently used by the group of patients of interest. This approach is being used by several health authorities and simply attempts to estimate current expenditure and activity by disease, care setting or locality. Combined with information from needs assessment and audit, this is important for accountability and providing information that may highlight anomalies or possible options for change. A programme budget (and information from needs assessment) is most useful when little is known about how a service is currently provided. However, as with burden of disease studies, programme budgeting should not by itself be used for priority setting.

There are two main types of programme budgeting: "macro" and "micro". "Macro" programme budgeting attempts to classify total health authority expenditure by disease, care setting and locality by reorganising existing accounting and activity data.[8] Although one might think that such information is fundamental to running and managing a health authority, it is being used in only a handful of health boards and authorities. "Micro" programme budgeting attempts to estimate expenditure (and activity) within a particular "programme" of care, such as maternity services or child health services.[9,10] There are various ways to define a programme budget. Expenditure and activity can be defined by subprogramme (such as type of delivery for maternity care), by locality, or by care setting (for example, primary or secondary care). When the programme budget can be defined in many ways, a flow chart can be used showing patients' pathways through care from the initial point of contact, and activity and expenditure identified at each stage.[11]

Both approaches (micro and macro) can also be applied at the level of a general practice, although there are few examples of where this has occurred.[12] Table 8.1 shows an example of a "micro" programme budget for asthma in a total fundholding pilot site of two general practices. Information on activity was obtained from patients' notes and details of the study can be found elsewhere.[12] This classified expenditure and activity by type of contact and by practice.

Table 8.1   Programme budget for asthma: costs (and activity)* (1995/1996)

| | Nairn (n = 565) | Ardersier (n = 226) | Total (n = 791) | % of total cost |
|---|---|---|---|---|
| GP consultations | £4555 (538) | £3056 (361) | £7612 (900) | 25 |
| Practice nurse visits | £162 (73) | £0 (0) | £162 (73) | 0.5 |
| Hospital admissions | £2252 (5) | £0 (0) | £2252 (5) | 7 |
| Out-patient visits† | £4370 (74) | £1972 (47) | £6342 (120) | 21 |
| Home visits | £599 (16) | £250 (7) | £849 (22) | 3 |
| Prescribing | £10 147 | £3373 | £10 147 | 44 |
| Total cost | £22 086 | £8651 | £30 737 | |
| (cost per patient) | (£38.01) | (£38.28) | (£38.09) | |

* Figures may not add up exactly because of rounding.
† These activity figures are the total number of visits. Only a proportion of these were paid for since only a patient's first visit incurs a financial cost. An estimated 12 visits were paid for in Nairn (that is, 11.5 × £380 = £4370) and five in Ardersier.

## Evaluating options for change: marginal analysis and economic evaluation

The second stage of needs assessment is the evaluation of options for change. This is where the economic approach is most useful and most widely applied. Most needs assessments and associated decisions are made within a fixed budget. Therefore any service expansions have to be counterbalanced by contraction or withdrawal of services elsewhere. In more formal economic evaluation, however, the options may be more obvious (for example, two alternatives within a trial). The economic framework contributes to the evaluation process by trying to ensure that the overall effect is to increase benefits from a given budget, and ensuring that benefits given up from reductions in activity are kept at a minimum. On the assumption that proposals for more resources (that is, investments) are effective, this involves answering two questions:

(1) Are there any current services which could be provided to the same level of effectiveness but with less resources, so freeing up some resources to implement some investments?

(2) If the answer to (1) is "no", are there some existing services which, despite being effective, are less effective per pound spent than some of the proposed investments?

89

In attempting to maximise the need met from a given amount of resources, some services that are effective will lose resources to other services that are more effective per pound spent. In so doing, overall effectiveness (that is, met need) will be maximised.

The economic framework can be applied comprehensively or pragmatically. The comprehensive approach is where economic evaluation is usually conducted as part of clinical trials and evaluations funded by long term research grants. It involves the measurement of resource use in each arm of a trial and also the measurement of consequences (that is, benefits to patients) in terms of measures of clinical effectiveness, life years saved, quality of life, and quality adjusted life years (QALYs). [13,14]

The pragmatic application of the economic framework recognises that it is impossible to conduct a randomised trial and detailed evaluation of resource use every time a decision is made by a purchaser about expanding or contracting health care services. The pragmatic approach, while still using the framework in the box above, uses information on costs from existing local data and makes "best guess" assumptions about how the use of resources is likely to change after an option is introduced.[7] Thus, the pragmatic approach can be conducted *before* the change has actually taken place. Evidence about changes in benefits to patients is obtained through literature reviews and the use of evidence based medicine. If there is no evidence, judgements have to be made. Even where few data are available, using the economic principles of opportunity cost and marginal analysis, specifying the alternatives clearly and merely listing the expected changes in resource use and benefits to patients may help to clarify many of the issues and value judgements involved.

For example, the margin identified for the case of asthma care in a general practice was the introduction of an asthma clinic.[12] The pragmatic approach used data from the literature to make assumptions about how the use of resources was likely to change if a clinic were introduced. These data were applied to the programme budget and several options for change were costed. Information on benefits to patients was obtained from the literature, where it was found that the evidence was not sufficient to say that an asthma clinic would improve or worsen the health of patients, although it may improve access.[15] It was therefore assumed that benefits to patients would be no worse. Two scenarios for an asthma clinic are shown in Table 8.2, where the marginal analysis examined the

Table 8.2   Marginal analysis of the introduction of an asthma clinic

|  | Nairn: 1 initial visit plus 2 follow-up visits for all asthmatics with a 50% attendance rate: costs (and number of contacts) | Ardersier: 1 initial visit plus 3 follow-up visits for 75% of asthmatics with a 50% attendance rate: costs (and number of contacts) |
|---|---|---|
| GP consultations | £2323 (275) | £1933 (228) |
| Practice nurse visits | £4862 | £1840 |
| Hospital admissions | £2252 (5) | £0 (0) |
| Out-patient visits | £1442 (3.8) | £981 (3) |
| Home visits | £240 (6) | £225 (6) |
| Prescribing | £10 451 | £3474 |
| Total cost | £21 571 | £8403 |
| Change in cost (total cost in programme budget minus total cost above) | −£514 | −£248 |

likely change in the value of resources from the introduction of an asthma clinic.

## Comprehensive versus pragmatic application of the economic framework

When comparing the comprehensive and pragmatic forms of economic evaluation, the latter may be criticised because of its perceived poor quality. In the pragmatic form, local data may be of poor quality (if there are data at all) which may hinder a firm conclusion about whether an option should go ahead. When the usefulness of the economic framework, however, is examined, the pragmatic should not only be compared with the comprehensive, but also with no economic evaluation at all. Compared with doing nothing or making decisions as before, using the economic framework in a simple way makes value judgments more explicit. It may also help to organise the available information in a way helpful to the decisions being made, and may be better than having no such information at all.

When you are judging the usefulness of the economic framework, it is important to bear in mind that, whether comprehensive or pragmatic, it does not remove the need for value judgements to be made. For example, if a randomised trial finds that a new service is likely to produce greater benefits but also incur greater costs, then a value judgment must be made as to whether the extra benefits are worth the extra costs. Neither form of evaluation will give you a yes/no answer and to assume that they do is naive. The economic framework outlined in this chapter (and indeed most forms of health care evaluation) should be used as an *aid* to decision making, rather than as a substitute for it.

## Conclusions

This chapter has outlined the argument that "needs assessment needs economics". Meeting health needs requires scarce resources which have alternative, perhaps more beneficial, uses. Use of the economic framework, either in a comprehensive or pragmatic way, should be integral to health needs assessments whether conducted at a national, health board, or general practice level. General

---

**Summary points**

- Economics tries to match needs met to resources available.
- To maximise the amount of need that can be met by limited resources, it is necessary to know:
  - the amount of need met by a health care intervention (effectiveness);
  - the resources used in meeting this need (cost).
- This involves:
  - examining how resources are currently used;
  - defining options for change (disinvestments as well as investments);
  - measuring the changes in costs and benefits of each option identified.
- The economic framework can be applied comprehensively (for example, economic evaluation alongside a randomised trial) or pragmatically in a purchasing context (for example, programme budgeting and marginal analysis combined with evidence from the literature).
- Although the comprehensive is preferred to the pragmatic, the pragmatic is better than no economic framework at all.

---

practitioners and public health professionals conducting needs assessments should enlist the advice of a local health economist, especially where options for change need to be identified and evaluated.

## Acknowledgements

Thanks to Shelley Farrar for comments on an earlier draft. The Health Economics Research Unit is funded by the Chief Scientist Office of the Scottish Office Department of Health. The views in this paper are those of the authors and not the Scottish Office Department of Health.

## References

1 Donaldson C, and Mooney G. Needs assessment, priority setting and contracts for health care: an economic view. *BMJ* 1991;**303**:1529–30.

2 Cohen D. Marginal analysis in practice: an alternative to needs assessment for contracting health care. *BMJ* 1994;**309**:781–5.

3 Donaldson C, Ratcliffe J, eds. Economics, public health and health care purchasing: reinventing the wheel? *Health Policy* 1995:**33**(2). Special issue.

4 Shiell A, Gerard K, Donaldson C. Cost of illness studies: an aid to decision making? *Health Policy* 1987;**8**:317–23.

5 Donaldson C. Purchasing to meet need. In: Culyer AJ, Wagstaff A, eds. *Reforming health care systems. Experiments with the NHS.* Proceedings of Section F (Economics) of the British Association for the Advancement of Science, 1994. Cheltenham: Edward Elgar; 1996.

6 Bryan S, Parkin D, Donaldson C. Chiropody and the QALY: a case study in assigning categories of disability and distress to patients. *Health Policy* 1991;**18**: 169–85.

7 Donaldson C, Walker A, Craig N. *Programme budgeting and marginal analysis. A handbook for applying economics in health care purchasing.* Glasgow Scottish Needs Assessment Programme, Scottish Forum for Public Health Medicine; 1995.

8 Miller P, Parkin D, Craig N, Lewis D, Gerard K. Less fog on the Tyne? Programme budgeting in Newcastle and North Tyneside. *Health Policy* 1997; **40**:217–29.

9 Ratcliffe J, Donaldson C, Macphee S. Programme budgeting and marginal analysis: a case study of maternity services. *J Public Health Medicine* 1996:**18**: 175–82.

10 Ruta D, Donaldson C, Gilray I. Economics, public health and health care purchasing: the Tayside experience. *J Health Services Research and Policy* 1996; **1**:185–93.

11 Posnett J, Street A. Programme budgeting and marginal analysis: an approach to priority setting in need of refinement. *J Health Services Research and Policy* 1996;**1**:147–153

12 Scott A, Currie N, Donaldson C, Wordsworth S. *A PBMA of asthma and diabetes care in the Nairn and Ardersier total fundholding pilot site. Report to*

*Grampian Health Board.* University of Aberdeen: Health Economics Research Unit, 1996.

13 Robinson R. Economic evaluation in health care. What does it mean? *BMJ* 1993;**307**:670–3.

14 Donaldson C, Shackley P. Economic evaluation. In: Detels R, Holland WW, McEwen J, Omenn GS, eds. *Oxford textbook of public health* 3rd ed. *Volume 2: The Methods of Public Health.* Oxford: Oxford University Press; 1997.

15 Eastwood AJ, Sheldon TA. Organisation of asthma care: what difference does it make? A systematic review of the literature. *Quality in Health Care* 1996;**5**: 134–43.

# Index